TODAY'S CHOICES. TOMORROW'S HEALTH:

Small steps to improve health, food choices, exercise, and life

By Dr. Justin Trosclair, D.C.

Inspired by Dr. Trevor VanWyk, D.C.
Edited by: Dr. Emer Garry

Special thanks to Dr. Trevor VanWyk, D.C. for the inspiration on some of the topics in this book. Your emails have been truly valuable and a catalyst for the creation of this book.

This work is dedicated to my wife, JingJing Zhao. I cherish you and can't thank you enough for being so supportive, among all the other things I love about you.

Copyright © 2017 Text by Dr. Justin Trosclair, D.C.

All rights reserved. No part of this book may be reproduced in any form or by any electronic, mechanical, or other means without prior permission in writing from the publisher.

Disclaimer:

This book is meant to provide general information about health subjects and health strategies. It should not be used as sole guidance for making healthcare decisions. The content within is not written as final medical or personal advice. I am not your doctor. This information is not intended as healthcare advice. This work is provided without express or limited warranty of any kind by either the author or anyone who has been involved in the creation, production, or distribution of this report. This includes, but is not limited to, the implied warranties of fitness for a particular purpose. The determination of the risk and usability of the information contained herein rests entirely with the reader. Dr. Justin Trosclair, editors and the final publisher of this book recommend that you seek a qualified and experienced professional when implementing any type of healthcare advice or changes, especially about food and exercise. The publisher and author assume no responsibility or warranties or guarantees of any kind for any errors or omissions. In no case shall the author be held responsible for any loss or other damages caused by the use and misuse of, or inability to use, any or all of the information described in this report. The information within this book represents the views of the author at the date of publication. Due to the rapid increase in knowledge, the author reserves the right to update and modernize his views as science uncovers more information. While every attempt has been made to verify the information, the author cannot accept responsibility for inaccuracies or oversights. Any perceived disrespect against organizations or individual persons is unintentional. The author makes no guarantee or warranty pertaining to the success of the reader using this material. By taking legal possession of this document you agree to these terms. If this agreement is violated, you will be notified via certified mail to cease and desist the use of this campaign; you will lose your lifetime right to use this material for your own personal use.

Reproduction of Material:

This book should not be reprinted, emailed, faxed, sold, copied, or distributed to others in any way. Consider the information in this book as copyrighted just like any book you would buy. Digital and print books have the same legal rights. Please don't commit illegal sharing. Even if you received this book free from some kind of promotion from me, you paid for it by giving me a valid email address. I expect the same from other readers. If you are a doctor or someone else that bought my book (actually paid for it with currency), you can resell it and make a markup. Thank you for being honest.

It is my hope that doctors and others will find value in the book and purchase it. For yourself, maybe to give to your patients as a gift or just have people buy it from you with a markup. With that said, please respect the effort it takes to write a book of any caliber and don't email this to others or print if off for others. What you can do is share with them the following website www.adoctorperspective.net or www.drjustintrosclair.com and look for the book link. You can also go to online book stores and buy it there too.

Exclusive Access

As a special thank you for buying this book, you have special access to the exclusive Facebook group "Today's Choices Tomorrows Health". www.facebook.com/groups/1869613209971935 Just send a request with the following code "**Step By Step**" and gain full access to a community of readers like yourself for support, questions and motivation.

ABOUT THE AUTHOR

Dr. Justin Trosclair is a practicing doctor of chiropractic and obtained his degree from the Texas Chiropractic College in Pasadena, TX with academic honors. He was born and raised in the heart of Cajun Country, Louisiana and received a Bachelor of Science from Louisiana State University. Dr. Justin spent almost seven years practicing in a suburb of Denver, Colorado before working in Yunnan, China for 3 years. As of the writing of this book, 2017, he is still residing in China working at a hospital. Dr. Trosclair is also the host of "A Doctor's Perspective" podcast where he interviews doctors and guests about success, overcoming obstacles, marketing, entertainment and how to have an optimal home-life balance. Please visit www.adoctorsperspective.net to listen and why not subscribe so you never miss an episode or other announcements. His personal clinic website can be found at www.drjustintrosclair.com. Dr. Justin is happily married to an amazing Christian woman, JJ for short. He can't say enough good things about JJ and would feel remiss if he left any out. Dr. Trosclair is available for interviews, guest speaking, and many other opportunities, so just reach out. He can be contacted at justin@adoctorsperspective.net

INTRODUCTION

First, I want to say a quick thank you for picking up this book. It's my sincere hope that you learn at least one thing from it and that you take actionable steps to go along with that new knowledge. Some of the topics may seem a bit controversial and some will resonate with you perfectly. You may scratch your head and say, "I never thought about it that way, but yeah I guess it makes sense." I do think a few of these chapters will challenge the way you typically think about what health really is. Change is up to you.

Who am I? My name is Dr. Justin Trosclair, Doctor of Chiropractic. I was born and raised in South Louisiana, attended Louisiana State University and then studied chiropractic in Houston at the Texas Chiropractic College. Immediately after graduation, I took over a failing private practice in Colorado and over the next 6-7 years worked on growing it and growing myself. Marketing and networking lessons were learned, best practices for patient outcomes were fine-tuned, and figuring out how to be an entrepreneur in the realm of healthcare was and is constantly evolving. My priorities slowly started changing and I decided to sell that clinic and move to China to work in a private hospital. I have now been the sole chiropractor in a small town of 200,000 people for 3 years. My profession is not even on the study curriculum in China so they hire some of us to integrate with the Traditional Chinese Medicine (TCM) departments. In fact, I am one of the two chiropractors in my entire province. During my chiropractic education and career I could have become certified in acupuncture and implemented it in my American practice but at the time I didn't know enough about acupuncture to invest my time and energy. Here in China, acupuncture is mainstream and in just about every hospital. If you were to look at our TCM department, you would say it sure looks similar to an integrated chiropractic or physical therapy clinic here in the States.

Now back to this book. Over the years, patients tend to ask the same questions. I also tend to have the same answers for those questions as well as my own education that I think will benefit them. At times, the concepts and paradigm shifts can be controversial, tough to swallow or easy to digest (depends on the person), take too much time to explain, or the topics aren't easily fit into a conversation with a patient in a natural way. No one who comes to a clinic in pain wants to hear a long speech about how chiropractic is different or how all the research proves what we are doing or how it is not only a safe alternative to medical care (for similar conditions) but it also beats it in certain situations. In fact, you may not even want to read a book about it either. I challenge you to approach the first third of this book with an open mind. Even if you have a negative view on chiropractic, the stories and examples still hold true and you could translate the lessons outlined into your own story and life. If I were an auto mechanic trying to explain these new health paradigms, I would use mechanic stories because that's what I would be intimately familiar with... but I'm not a mechanic.

It's important to realize that some topics are just easier to understand when we use examples. Why is pain a good thing? Just because you feel fine, does that mean you don't have anything wrong with you? Why does a person go to a chiropractor for a few weeks versus just once to the medical doctor? Why is it important to be aware of the types of food you eat and understand what's actually healthy? Is portion control and moderation even doable because I've tried before and failed? Exercise tips, hacks, and answering the question, "what's right for me and my condition" need to be examined as well. All these topics will be addressed in this book. Stories, examples and relating issues to a concept or profession someone is already acquainted with is how this book will be laid out. It should bridge the unknown and unfamiliar with topics you already understand to be true.

The content of this book was originally in the form of blog posts on my clinic website aimed at exploring in more detail the questions, answers and topics previously mentioned. Some of the selected posts were the most read and others were ones I felt important to share in this format. I edited some of the content and flow so it reads more like a book than a website asking for clicks, become a patient and whatnot. As mentioned, I am a chiropractor so the first part of the book is going to be written with health mindsets and patient concerns that I came across with my professional view. The beauty of it is that the principles are still true and if you pause and reflect on what was written, you can learn something for yourself as well, even if you don't like my profession. I will also go over some basic food concepts and how to make healthier choices. Lastly, I cover some real world tips and actual exercises so you can better stabilize your spine and strengthen your muscles. The goal is for you to be able to implement something today and start making better choices for your well-being. Let's focus on real health care and preventative actions versus only dealing with issues when they arise and using doctors when we are sick.

Feel free to skip around the book chapters. Each chapter stands alone, so read what interests you most first. I go on laser-focused rants and health hack nuggets of information throughout the book. I encourage you to read the whole book because you never know if an ill-placed hack will be just what you need to make those incremental steps for lifelong health. Throughout the book you will see bold text, highlighted boxes, and other ways to grab your attention to what I feel are the biggest, most helpful hacks that your Momma just never knew to tell you about.

Again, I want to thank you for the trust in getting this book. I want to respect your time and make positive changes in your mind and body. I welcome questions, concerns, positive testimonies and the like: so please contact me.

I have a podcast called A Doctor's Perspective where I interview other doctors and guests and find out what successes they have had, struggles they have endured and overcome, practice management tips, marketing and how to not just balance work and family life but to excel at family life. You can contact me via email at justin@adoctorsperspective.net and I look forward to connecting with you on my Facebook of Dr Justin, of the podcast's Facebook page, Twitter, Instagram, Pinterest and Flickr.

Have a great day and enjoy!

TABLE OF CONTENTS

About the Author i

Introduction ii

1. How Does Your Body Work 1
2. The Cause of Interference 5
3. The 5 Ways Subluxations Occur: Spinal Misalignments 8
4. Does Pain Have Any Redeeming Benefits? 11
5. Why Some People Are Negative About Chiropractic ... 14
6. Secret Research from 1921 is Finally Revealed 18
7. New Information on How You Can Improve Your Health 21
8. Are You Minimizing? 25
9. Can Your Body Heal Itself? 27
10. Do You Want To Be Sick? 29
11. How Perception Alters Your Reality 32
12. Doc, Do What You Did Last Time 34
13. Study Shows How to Get More Out Of Chiropractic ... 37
14. Work Injury Recovery and With Fewer Surgery: Sign Me Up 39
15. Blueprint to Reboot your Nervous System: Chiropractic Summary 41
16. The 5 Essential Habits of Great Health + 6 Bonuses ... 47

    Two Simple Changes to Your Plate that Fool Your Hunger Meter 50

Lesson Learned Living in China 52

Secret Chinese Pepper Flake Oil Recipe 53

When It's Food Time, Don't Sit In Front of Electronics 54

Be Mindful of When and How You Eat 54

Two Tidbits about Consistency and Long-Term Goals 56

17. The Truth About Fat in your Diet 59

18. New Concept: Ketogenic Based Diets 61

    Extra Tidbit: Sugar Creates Inflammation 62

    Word of Caution: Why Am I so Grumpy When Off the Carbs? 64

    Secret Hack: Don't Let Fake Sugar Fake You Out 64

    Bonus Tip about Sugar Alcohols 65

19. 5 Quick Steps to Mastering Food Labels 67

20. Being Hungry and Dealing with It 71

21. Better to Eat More at Breakfast, Lunch or Dinner 74

22. Understanding Organic Food Labels 75

23. When is The Best Time to Exercise? 77

24. Testosterone and How to Maximize it for Exercise 78

25. Personal Blueprint - Cardio: 80

26. Personal Blueprint - Weightlifting 83

27. Weight Lift Booster and Schedule: 86

28. Personalized Calorie Consumption Calculator 88

    Time to Break Out your Calculators and Find Your Calorie Goals 92

Calculating the Three Formulas for Optimal Calorie Consumption 95

    Step 2: Activity Multiplier 96

    Step 3: Slow Drop in Calories and Macronutrient Ratios 99

    Gradual Reduction of Calories Method 101

Macronutrient Ratios 103

    What is a Macronutrient? 104

    Tools to Help 109

Intermittent Fasting Guide 113

    16/8 Fast 115

    24-Hour Fast 116

29. Make This Simple Change In Your Exercise For Better Results 119

30. Are 20 Minute Workouts Any Good 121

31. Cardio Health Hack: Interval Training: 122

32. Exercises to Help You Reduce Neck and Shoulder Pain .. 124

33. Bonus Idea for the Shoulder - Rotator Cuff 128

34. 3 Easy Exercises to Tone Your Stomach 130

35. Bonus Exercise: Sucking in the Gut versus Hollowing the Abdominals 133

36. Exercises to Help Strengthen the Low Back and the Unknown Core Muscles 135

37. A Quick and Easy Stretch for Back Pain Sufferers and Desk Workers 139

38. When Should I Stretch? 141

39. What are Nerve Glide/ Flossing Stretches and How They Stop Numbness in the Arms and Legs 143

Basics of how nerves travel in the body and why they can get injured 143

What are Adhesions? 144

What are Nerve Flossing Stretches? 145

Low Back and Leg Numbness & Tingling 146

    Stretch for Disc Bulges 146

    Sciatic Nerve 147

Neck and Arm and Hand Numbness & Tingling 148

    Start Here: Top 3 Stretches 148

    Median Nerve 149

    Radial Nerve 149

    Ulnar Nerve 150

40. Bonus: 6 Ways to Eliminate Headaches Before They Start 151

41. Hidden Ergonomic Tip: Stop the 3pm Headache? 154

42. Bonus: Study Shows Lost Sleep Cannot Be Made Up 155

43. Making a Budget 158

    Cheap vs. Frugal 164

    The Value of Relationships and Money 166

How did I overspend so much? Now what? 171

    STEP 1: Gathering the Information 171

Phase 2 of Step 1: Write it down 175

    Gather your paychecks for the last three months 176

- Write down your expenses 177
- No lumping together, Point 1 178
- Point 2 179
- Method 1: Broken down correctly with receipts 180
- Method 2: Guessing the amount you spent based on a percentage because you only have grand totals 180
- New Month- Current Day to Day Bills. 181
- STEP 2: Compare Income vs. Expenses 181
- STEP 3: Evaluate Overspending and Reduce It 187

Basics on Retirement 217
- Roth IRA 220
- Traditional IRA 221
- 401K/ Simple IRA 221
- Trust Fund 221
- Buying Houses 222
- Rapid Compounding Debt Payoff 223

44. Conclusion 226

1 HOW DOES YOUR BODY WORK

I've found that patients who have a general idea of how their body works get better results with their care and heal faster. So let me give you the two-minute version.

Do you know what controls all the activities within your body? How does your heart beat? How does your stomach digest food? How does your body create new cells? What's making all this happen? If you answered blood, heart or our cardiovascular system then you guessed wrong, like 70% of the people. Now, I'm not saying you can survive without your heart beating or if you lose too much blood, but there is another system in our body that is even more important because without it working properly your heart can stop beating altogether. The correct answer is the nervous system.

The nervous system is the master control system of the body. In Grey's Anatomy textbook it says, *The nervous system controls and coordinates all organs and structures of the human body*. The nervous system is made up of the brain, spinal cord and all of the nerves that travel throughout the body. For your body to be healthy and work properly, your brain has to be able to communicate with the rest of the body without any problems.

Your brain communicates with your body through the nerves.

As long as your brain can send information to your body via these nerves without any problems, your body will function normally. However, if there is anything interfering with the brain's ability to communicate with your body, or your body's ability to communicate with the brain, then there's going to be a problem. In other words, if something interferes with the nerve pathways between the brain and to the body, there will be consequences. The body will start to malfunction. Your organs, tissues and structures will not be at 100% and you will develop pain, symptoms or other serious health problems over time.

Let me give you an example.

Do you know who Christopher Reeve is? He was the actor who played Superman in the original movies. Unfortunately, he suffered a great tragedy during a hobby he loved...riding horses. In May of 1995, during the cross-country portion of an event in Culpeper, Virginia, Reeve's thoroughbred, Eastern Express, balked at a rail jump and pitched his rider forward. Reeve's hands were tangled in the horse's bridle and he landed head first, fracturing the uppermost bones in his neck. The injury to his spine had caused so much trauma to the spinal cord and spinal nerves that he instantly became paralyzed. Later, the doctors determined that Reeve's brain was working perfectly...it just wasn't able to send information to or receive information from the rest of the body because of the damage to the spinal cord.

Do you see what happens when the brain is unable to communicate with the rest of the body? I've shown you that if the nerve pathways are damaged badly enough they can cause paralysis, but what else can it cause?

When adults have nerve interference, it can cause back pain, neck pain, headaches, stomach trouble, fatigue, depression, muscle spasm and tension, numbness, tingling, loss of strength, loss of flexibility and the list goes on. It can cause hundreds of symptoms and areas of malfunction in the body. When there's a problem with the nerve pathways in children, it may contribute to ear infections, colic, bedwetting, reflux, fatigue and pain, to name a few. In practice we see a lot of these problems get better in kids but the research is still catching up.

As soon as there's interference in the nerve "communication" pathways, the body will malfunction. It's important that you know you could feel great and be completely unaware that your body is malfunctioning. Almost every disease or health problem in the body always starts off painlessly. There are people who have been given a clean bill of health at the doctor's office and have died of a fatal heart attack a week later. Diabetes, tooth cavities and cancer are three other examples that are slow to show symptoms. If you don't get blood work done every year, you will be unaware that you are on your way to no longer being able to eat all the sugar you want. If we catch it early, we can change our diet and exercise more, maybe even add some supplements and then reverse the damage that has accumulated. Oftentimes, we develop odd pains in our abdomen or in a joint, finally go to the doctor, a scan is performed, and you discover that cancer has been growing inside you for 2 years and has only started to cause pain because of how big it has become.

I say all this because many people might know this subconsciously, but it's not until somebody verbalizes it in a way that is easily understood that they connect all the dots. A malfunction in the body starts off painlessly. Don't assume that just because you feel good you don't have interference to your nerve system. You know what else starts out painless? Spinal Problems.

Let's summarize:

**The nervous system controls and coordinates all the organs and structures of the body.

**If there is any interference or damage to the nerve pathways, the body will start to malfunction. You cannot have nerve interference and optimal health.

**Your nervous system is the most important system in your body so you need to take care of it on a regular basis as you age.

2 THE CAUSE OF INTERFERENCE

You just learned that your nervous system (brain, spinal cord and nerves) is the most important system in the human body. It's the communication network that controls every cell, tissue and organ, and keeps everything working properly. Any interference to this system will cause your body to malfunction. When your body malfunctions, it's near impossible to have optimal health.

Now I want to share with you what the #1 cause of interference to your nervous system is: a condition called subluxation. A subluxation occurs when there is a misalignment or a loss of motion of one or more of the bones in the spine, causing a problem with the nerve(s) in that area. Medically speaking, a subluxation is almost a dislocation of a joint and that is not what I am referring to here. The way I like to describe a subluxation is by calling this condition a spinal misalignment. The vertebrae are experiencing a lack of motion because of trauma, wear and tear, tight muscles, ligaments and tendons that are inflamed or otherwise injured and this can cause pain, tenderness, numbness, suboptimal nervous system health and, for many people, no symptoms at all for many years to decades (their spine may suffer arthritis, but I'm jumping ahead of myself).

Subluxations create interference to the nerve signals, causing the body to malfunction. They destroy the ability of the brain and body to properly communicate with one another, resulting in a loss of health. They can have devastating effects on your quality of life. When the nervous system is malfunctioning because of spinal subluxations, normal communication pathways are interrupted and the nervous system no longer has the ability to function properly. It's usually not an immediate malfunction and most of the time for most of people the impairment will be below a conscious level. Research has actually shown, though, with the elderly and with athletes, that fine motor skills and overall performance are increased with faster recovery when subluxations are removed.

Your body performs worse at every level. Your immune system weakens, your strength and coordination are negatively affected, your emotional state can be altered, your organs may not function normally and you could experience a constant state of pain, stiffness, lack of flexibility, stress, fatigue and many other symptoms. Did you know that almost all professional sports teams have someone on staff to help rid them of subluxations? It's true, and those who use it notice a difference in performance and recovery time. Peer-reviewed research studies also report the benefits of this. Subluxations, just like cavities, cancer and many other diseases, can start out PAINLESS. And if they are left uncorrected, they continue to get worse.

If you have areas in your spine that are subluxated, due to malfunctions in your nervous system, it's impossible for you to have optimal health. That's why having a healthy spine is so important.

==================================
Chiropractic procedures are the #1 option for the detection and correction of subluxations and nerve malfunction. This makes chiropractors unique.
==================================

I am a Doctor of Chiropractic and a chiropractor's job is to restore health to the areas of your spine that have subluxations. It's my job to make sure your nervous system is as healthy as possible. It's my job to not only get you out of pain when you hurt, but also keep your body as healthy as possible. And of course, I'm a little biased but the research backs us chiropractors up. There are myths and negative thoughts about us and I'll discuss why that is later in the book.

Let's summarize:

**The nervous system controls and coordinates all the organs and structures of the body.

**If there is any interference or damage to the nerve pathways, the body will eventually malfunction and health problems will result. You cannot have subluxations and optimal health.

**Subluxations destroy the ability of neurological networks to work properly, resulting in a loss of health. They can have devastating effects on your quality of life.

3 THE 5 WAYS SUBLUXATIONS OCCUR: SPINAL MISALIGNMENTS

You learned that a subluxation is when your spine is jammed or misaligned and causes an interference with the normal function of your nervous system. You also learned that subluxations cause your body to malfunction and not function normally.

A common question I get from new patients regarding subluxations is, "How does my spine get that way?"

The obvious answer is from trauma, like auto accidents, falls or any sudden physical injuries. There are also four "not so obvious" reasons why people lose the health in their spine and develop subluxations.

The first reason is everyday wear and tear. You see, most subluxations don't just suddenly show up. No, most subluxations develop over time. Little by little, our everyday activities start to wear down our spines and we start to develop subluxations over time.

The second reason is the aging process. As we get older, our bodies naturally start to break down and deteriorate. The aging process can cause arthritis, degeneration and subluxations in your spine.

The third reason is stress. There are three different types of stress that affect the health of your spine and body: physical stress, chemical stress and emotional stress. Stress has been proven to have negative effects on the body, including the spine. There's no question that most people live very fast paced stressful lives these days and stress causes subluxations.

The final reason is neglect. Over 80% of our population experiences back or neck pain or health problems as a result of spinal subluxations. Headaches, numbness in the arms or legs, disc bulges, pain with lying down or standing, discomfort when twisting and a host of other symptoms could be caused by unknown subluxations. It's very common for patients who have received treatment and are out of pain to begin to realize when their body is experiencing subluxations again. They might feel the tightness between the shoulders reappear or discomfort after standing for an hour instead of four and they recognize that a quick tune up will help these symptoms disappear again. Depending on the person, they might stay away for a few weeks, a few months or even a whole year.

The reason so many people suffer from subluxations is because most people don't take care of their spine. You wouldn't expect your car to run optimally if you never serviced it and took good care of it, would you? How about your teeth? What if you never brushed them? Do you think the chance of getting cavities increases? You bet.

The spine is no different. When you ignore taking care of your spine, everyday wear and tear, the aging process and stress will take their toll.

So let's summarize. Here are the five ways your spine can become unhealthy and develop subluxations.

1. Trauma
2. Everyday wear and tear
3. The aging process
4. Physical, chemical and emotional stress
5. Neglect

4 DOES PAIN HAVE ANY REDEEMING BENEFITS?

When it comes to health in America, what do most people focus on? That's right, pain. So what is pain? Pain is the warning signal from your body to let you know something's wrong. Let me illustrate what pain is with a story.

Let's say you are cooking dinner in your kitchen. The phone rings and when you answer it, you hear the voice of your best friend. You start chatting away and before you know it you've forgotten that you've got dinner cooking on the stove. All of a sudden you hear a loud blaring siren noise. You instantly realize it's your smoke alarm! You run into the kitchen and see a fire on the stove. Smoke is billowing everywhere! The smoke from the fire caused your smoke alarm to go off and alerted you that there's a fire in your kitchen. At this point, what do you do?

Well, one option would be to focus on putting out the fire. That seems like the most logical thing to do. What do you think? A second option would be to get out your ladder and turn off the smoke alarm. Don't worry about the fire; just get rid of that loud obnoxious noise. Would you choose the second option? Does it even make sense to turn off the smoke alarm and ignore the fire and let it continue to burn? Not really.

I hope you'd focus on putting out the fire. The only reason the smoke alarm is even making noise in the first place is because of the fire. So we have a cause (the fire) and an effect (the smoke alarm going off). Wouldn't you solve BOTH problems by putting out the fire? If you put out the fire, you no longer have a fire and you also don't have a smoke alarm blaring. Make sense?

Now let's go back to learning about pain. Like I said before, pain is your body's warning signal that something is wrong. It's a signal, just like the smoke alarm. Unfortunately, when it comes to health, people make the mistake of focusing only on their pain and not what's causing it. If it doesn't make sense to turn off the smoke alarm and leave the fire burning, it shouldn't make sense to focus only on the pain either. Pain is an effect. It always has a cause.

And here's the secret I want to share with you today: The people who have optimal health focus on healing THE CAUSE of their pain and symptoms. Read that again. It's extremely important.

When you focus on healing the cause of pain, you not only get rid of the pain that's bugging you, you also have a stronger and healthier body (which is something you should want!). If you only focus on the pain then you never really solve the most important problem. Your body will still have problems and your pain will most likely come back. Does this make sense?

Is pain a bad thing? Most people think it is but I disagree. Pain is very helpful. Without feeling pain, how would you know something was wrong with your body? What about being pain-free? If we don't have pain, are we healthy? Not necessarily. There are many diseases and health problems that begin in your body without pain. Cancer, high blood pressure and back problems are just a few. Often, by the time you feel pain, the disease or health problem is not a new problem...it's advanced.

So remember these two things:
1. Make the commitment to heal the CAUSE of your pain. It's a better choice.
2. Take care of yourself even when you feel good. Health problems may be developing even when you are pain-free.

5 WHY SOME PEOPLE ARE NEGATIVE ABOUT CHIROPRACTIC

This section is a little longer, but I promise it will be worth your time. I want to share with you the truth about what happened to the chiropractic profession.

I've got a question for you...Do you know anyone who doesn't "believe" in chiropractic care? You know the people who say things like..."Chiropractors aren't real doctors," "I don't believe in chiropractors," "I would never go to a chiropractor." I'm sure you've heard these kinds of comments before. They may even be coming from family members, friends, or co-workers. As a joke, I like to counter this sometimes with, "I'm not the Easter bunny or the tooth fairy. I'm real. I'm standing in front of you. There's nothing to believe in." Of course, that's a bit sarcastic and I know what they mean. Let's continue on our journey, shall we?

========================
Why People Think This Way
========================

Chances are pretty good that your opinion about chiropractic is favorable. Patients consistently rate satisfaction of their chiropractor at 95% and these favorable results for back and neck pain are statistically significant. But what about the people who are negative about chiropractic care? Have you ever wondered WHY these people feel this way? After all, you know how beneficial chiropractic is...how safe it is... how it makes you feel better and improves your health. Even though chiropractic care is as popular as ever today, it wasn't always that way. So let's go over what caused people to have a negative perception about chiropractic care.

Disclaimer: I am not one of the chiropractors who disapprove of all medical doctors and bash them and think patients should never take drugs. In fact, I have healthy relationships with medical doctors and believe in the medical profession and that surgeries, drugs, etc do have their place. However, the following story remains true.

======================
The Guilty Party: The AMA
======================

The story goes something like this:

Back in the 1940's and the 1950's, chiropractic care was gaining in popularity across the United States and that was a big problem for the American Medical Association (AMA). You see, from a business perspective, the AMA viewed the chiropractic profession as a "threat" to the business of medicine. The American Medical Association opposes all forms of health care that cut into its profits. So in 1963, a committee was formed within the AMA called the committee on quackery. Their job? To "contain and eliminate" the chiropractic profession. Don't believe me? Check this out. In 1971, in a memo to the AMA Board of Trustees, Doyle Taylor said, "Your Committee has considered its prime mission to be the first containment of

Chiropractic and ultimately the elimination of Chiropractic." Let's keep going.

So this committee did three things in their efforts to destroy the chiropractic profession. First, they made it illegal for medical doctors who were members of the AMA to work with chiropractors. If a medical doctor was found working with a chiropractor, they were kicked out of the AMA. The second thing that happened was new medical doctors were taught in medical school that chiropractors were unscientific quacks and working with them was to be avoided. The third thing that happened is that, for over 20 years, this committee disseminated false information to the general public. They did it through the school systems, the press, through hospitals and doctors...you name it.

=================
The AMA Gets Sued
=================

In October of 1976, a chiropractor by the name of Dr. Chester Wilk and four other chiropractors sued the AMA. To make a long story short, in 1987, following 11 years of legal action, the AMA was found guilty. In 1987, Judge Susan Getzedanner, ruled that the AMA had engaged in an illegal conspiracy to destroy the chiropractic profession by engaging in "systematic, long-term wrong-doing with the long-term intent to destroy a licensed profession."

The AMA was ordered to cease and desist. Judge Getzedanner also ordered "a permanent injunction against the AMA," forcing them to print the court's findings in the Journal of the American Medical Association. This decision was upheld by the U.S. Supreme Court in 1990.

===========================
The Big Problem with All Of This
===========================

So now that you know the truth about what happened to the chiropractic profession, do you see the big problem here? Here it is: People who don't believe in chiropractic care have a belief system that is based on a lie created by the American Medical Association. This lie was PROVEN to be a lie at the Supreme Court level in our court system. And because of this lie, there are now millions of people in our country who believe something that isn't true.

Chiropractic has been a great profession THE ENTIRE TIME and it will continue to be a great profession.

What's worse is this: Think about the millions of people in our country suffering needlessly every day because they don't think chiropractic care is an option...because they were taught not to go to chiropractors. Do you know how many people would be healthier and would feel better if they knew the truth and started going to a chiropractor? It would be millions.

So please do me a favor. If you know someone who "doesn't believe" in chiropractic, share this story with them. Gently tell them that what they were taught was a lie...and that chiropractic care is a great way to get healthy and stay healthy. It's time to stop believing in lies and believing the truth.

6 SECRET RESEARCH FROM 1921 IS FINALLY REVEALED

Secret research from 1921 is finally being revealed. In 1921, a medical doctor by the name of Henry Windsor wanted to know if there was any connection between minor abnormal curvatures of the spine and diseased organs and whether an abnormal misalignment of the spine caused disease to the organs.

The Shocking Secret Dr. Windsor Discovered...Dr. Windsor used 50 cadavers from the University of Pennsylvania for his study. He discovered through his examination and studies that in 50 cadavers with disease in 139 organs, there was an abnormal misalignment of the spine that belonged to the same nerve segments as the diseased organs almost 100% of the time.

Dr. Windsor discovered there was a direct link between spinal misalignments and diseased organs. In his research conclusions, Dr. Windsor stated the following: "It was rare to find an organ with disease which was not supplied by the same nerves as the vertebrae with misalignment."

The misalignments of the spine preceded organ disease. Spinal misalignment appears to precede old age and causes it. The spine becomes unhealthy first and disease and old age follows.

But has the research from 1921 stood the test of time? You may be wondering if there is any current research to validate the work done over 80 years ago by Dr. Windsor. That's a fair question...one that I had myself, and after a little digging the answer is YES.

In a study published in September 2005, a group of medical doctors and Ph.D.s were trying to determine if poor posture of the neck and upper back caused an increase in the poor health and mortality (death) rate in older populations. The medical doctors studied 1,353 people to assess this. Can you guess what they found???

The doctors found that with increasing misalignment and poor posture, there was a trend towards greater mortality (death). They also concluded that poor posture in the neck and upper back was significantly associated with deaths due to atherosclerosis. For deaths due to atherosclerosis, participants with poor posture in the neck and upper back had a significant 2.4 times greater death rate. Even mild misalignment and poor posture had a definite greater rate of earlier death. Poor posture and misalignment of the neck and upper back reflect an increased rate of aging.

=============
My Comments:
=============

Not much to say, except for the obvious: your spine plays a BIG role in your overall health. People who think the spine is a body part that can be neglected are making a huge mistake. People who take care of their teeth on a regular basis, yet never take care of their spine, are missing a big piece of the health and wellness puzzle. If it's scientifically proven that an unhealthy spine can contribute to pain, organ disease and early death, don't you think it's a good idea to keep your spine healthy? Take action - get healthy - stay healthy

7 NEW INFORMATION ON HOW YOU CAN IMPROVE YOUR HEALTH

I've come across some exciting new research you're definitely going to want to know about. A landmark study done by researchers at the University of Lund found that chiropractic care positively influences overall health. This means that chiropractic care is PROVEN to do more than just treat aches and pains.

Here's what the researchers found: As our bodies are subjected to physical, chemical and psychological stress, we develop what's called oxidative stress, which causes disease and accelerated aging. This fact is well known and accepted throughout the research community. Oxidative stress causes DNA damage and block DNA repair.

The study confirmed that chiropractic adjustments have a positive effect on the body at the cellular level and can help lower oxidative stress in the body. This study was published in the Journal of Vertebral Subluxation Research, and was also reported in Medical News Today.

==
Save Money and Improve Your Health With Chiropractic Care
==

The second exciting study was conducted at the Parker College of Chiropractic by Dr. Ron Rupert and his team of researchers. The study surveyed over 300 people, ages 65 years and older, who had received chiropractic care for 5 years or longer. They found that patients who received a chiropractic adjustment once a month for 5 years or longer spent only 31% of the national average for health care services when compared with US citizens of the same age. The patients receiving chiropractic care spent 69% LESS than what the average American spends on healthcare. The chiropractic patients also had 50% FEWER medical provider visits than the average Americans of the same age.

These benefits were not seen in patients who only used chiropractic for short-term care. That's why it's so important to take care of yourself on a regular basis. Now I don't know about you, but if you can save money and improve your health at the same time, that seems like a no-brainer to me!

Another study found that if you have low back pain and begin care with a doctor of chiropractic first, it will save you 40% on your healthcare costs when compared to starting with a medical doctor. The study reviewed data from 85,000 people with Blue Cross Blue Shield health insurance. It was also stated that insurance companies that restrict access to chiropractic care for low back pain treatment may pay more for care than they would if they offered chiropractic.

===

Chiropractic Improves the Health of Your Nervous System

===

The third study was done by John Zhang, M.D., Ph.D., and his team of researchers. They determined in their study that chiropractic care decreases pain and improves the function of the autonomic nervous system, which controls the organs, glands, and blood vessels.= This study is published in the Journal of Chiropractic Education, Vol. 2, No. 1, 2005.

What do these three studies have to do with the future of your health? The answer is "a lot." Healthcare in the United States is only going to get more and more expensive, it is estimated that one in every five dollars will be spent on your health by the year 2015. If you want to cut your costs on healthcare and give yourself the best chance possible to be healthy then research shows that regular chiropractic care is the answer.

Taking care of yourself on a regular, consistent basis is a huge responsibility. Taking care of your body regularly, and not just when you have pain, is a huge responsibility. Getting chiropractic adjustments on a regular basis is a huge responsibility. But it will pay off for you in two ways. You will save money on the costs of your healthcare as you get older and you will have better health overall. The investment of time and money is well worth it. Spend a little now or spend a lot more later.

Insanity is doing the same thing over and over and expecting a different result. If you want great health right now, if you want great health as you get older, then use services that will get you there. Chiropractic is scientifically proven to do that. This should be very exciting for you because now you know a PROVEN way to get healthy, stay healthy and save money on your healthcare as you get older.

So keep getting chiropractic care. The research says you'll have much better health and you'll save a ton of money if you do.

8 ARE YOU MINIMIZING?

There's a situation that comes up from time to time with my patients and people in general that I want to share with you. It's called minimizing. Let me illustrate what minimizing is with two stories.

The first story involves a female patient in her late 50's. She came into the office with severe lower back pain. Upon examination and X-ray, it was determined she had severe vertebral subluxations and advanced degeneration (arthritis) in her spine. Basically, her lower back was in BAD shape. There was a tremendous loss of health in that area of her body. This patient came in for her chiropractic adjustments for approximately two weeks and then stopped. I didn't see her until 2 months later. I asked her why she had stopped her care and her response was she didn't think the adjustments were working fast enough. She had returned because her pain was intensified and she had already gone through the conventional medical route which was not helping her and she was desperate.

The problem this patient had was she MINIMIZED the severity of her health problem, even after she'd been told how bad it was. Because she minimized her problem, she had an unrealistic expectation of how long it would take to feel better and restore health to her lower back to as near normal as possible. She didn't give herself enough time and chiropractic adjustments to heal the problem. Think about the last time you had a lung infection. We take a couple of pills three times a day for ten days. It took time and repetition for the pills and your body to destroy those harmful bacteria.

Here's the second story. A patient in her late 60's came into the office with terrible neck and shoulder pain. For her age, her spine wasn't great, but it wasn't terrible either. Each time this patient came in, she had an attitude of defeat. She would repeatedly say, "This is probably as good as I'll ever feel," or "I doubt I'll be able to get much better." This patient was minimizing her potential. This is very dangerous because when someone starts to give up hope and minimizes their ability to heal and be well, it is very hard to improve their level of health.

Ask yourself these two questions:

* Are you minimizing the reality of your current health?

* Are you minimizing your potential?

My suggestion is to not do either. Be real with yourself about your current health and make the commitment to do what it takes to get better and stay healthy. If you minimize your problem, you are not being honest with yourself.

This will set you up to be very frustrated because you think your problem will go away and be healed much faster than it really will. Never, and I mean NEVER, minimize your potential as a human being. You can accomplish great things, including improving your health, as long as you have the right attitude and commitment. If you minimize your potential, it becomes very hard to get what you truly want and desire.

9 CAN YOUR BODY HEAL ITSELF?

Is the human body capable of self-healing? Does your body have the ability to heal itself? Can your body heal naturally? Yes and no. Let me explain.

Your body definitely has the ability to heal itself naturally. For example, if you cut your finger, your body will mend and repair the wound. After several days the cut will be healed. However, sometimes the body is not able to heal all by itself. It needs some outside assistance. Take a broken bone, for example. If you break your arm, your body has the ability to heal the bone, but it doesn't have the ability to put the bone back into the correct position.

That's where a doctor comes in. A doctor puts the bone back into position and then the body heals itself. What about keeping your spine and nervous system healthy? When there are subluxations in the spine causing nerve interference, can the body heal itself or does it need some outside assistance? Subluxations and nerve interference need outside assistance to heal. That's what chiropractors are for!

Chiropractors assist your body in healing. Once the subluxations and nerve interference are removed, your body will function better and you will feel better. Make sense? Just remember that your body is incredibly powerful. It has the ability to heal naturally but sometimes needs a little assistance.

Removing subluxations and nerve interference is one of the health problems that the body cannot heal all by itself. That's why it's so important to get chiropractic adjustments to keep your spine healthy and free of subluxations because it's harder for your body to heal if there is nerve interference.

10 DO YOU WANT TO BE SICK?

I hope one of your top priorities in life is having great health because without great health NOTHING you do will be as enjoyable, productive or effective. So the question I have for you is, "What is health?" Most people answer that question by saying, "Health is feeling good." With this definition, if a person "feels good" then they must be healthy, right? The truth is health is much more than just feeling good.

The World Health Organization defines health as, "A state of optimal physical, mental and social well-being and not merely the absence of disease or infirmity. Webster's dictionary (www.m-w.com) defines health as, "The condition of being sound in body, mind or spirit."

Upon reading those definitions, it becomes pretty clear that health is not just how you feel, but rather how your mind and body are functioning.

Health = Function.

The next question I have is "Where does health come from?" Health comes from within you. Your body was designed to be able to heal itself naturally. Health is your natural state. Having constant pain, tight muscles, sickness or disease is not how we should be living. So why isn't everybody healthy? Great question. The answer is because we have ongoing physical, chemical and emotional stresses in our daily lives that slowly break our bodies down.

The aging process is also a destructive process that breaks our bodies down. We cannot escape the effects of aging. Just like a car that needs tune-ups and maintenance, our bodies need regular tune-ups and maintenance to keep the stress and aging from wearing us out. If you expect to enjoy great health as you get older, you have to take care of your body on a regular basis, otherwise aging and stress will continue to break your body down and wear it out, causing a ton of future health problems.

The last question I have is, "Do you want to be sick or do you want to be healthy?" It almost seems silly to be asking you this but I have a legitimate reason. The truth is no one ever tells me that they want to be sick or that they choose sickness over health...at least not with their words. However, when people do things they know are unhealthy, they are choosing to be sick...not with their words, but with their actions.

When people know they should exercise but don't, they are saying that they choose to move in the direction of sickness with their lack of action. People who know they should eat more nutritious foods because they have an unhealthy diet but don't change are moving in the direction of sickness. People who choose to smoke a pack of cigarettes a day are choosing sickness over health. Ask yourself, "Am I moving in the direction of sickness?" not with your words but with your actions or lack of actions?

What about being healthy? We choose to be healthy when we take actions that keep us healthy. When you do things like eat healthy foods, exercise, take time for prayer or meditation, get chiropractic adjustments, get massages, get enough rest and other healthy activities, you are moving in the direction of health...

...not just with words, with ACTIONS!

If you don't take a pro-active approach to your health and take advantage of products and services that create better health, your neglect will have a consequence...you move in the direction of sickness.

So I'll leave you with this question to think about in closing here: "What are some actions you can take on a more regular basis that will ensure you will be healthy and what are some things you can eliminate that are presently moving you towards being sick?"

11 HOW PERCEPTION ALTERS YOUR REALITY

A man came upon a construction site where three people were working. He asked the first, "What are you doing?" and the man answered, "I am laying bricks." He asked the second, "What are you doing?" and the man answered, "I am building a wall." He walked up to the third man, who was humming a tune as he worked, and asked, "What are you doing?" and the man stood and smiled and said, "I am building a cathedral."

Here's another story.

A man came upon a chiropractic office where three people were sitting in the reception room waiting to see the doctor. He asked the first, "What are you doing here?" and the man answered, "I am getting rid of my pain." He asked the second, "What are you doing here?" and the man answered, "I am correcting the cause of my pain and health problems." He walked over to a third person, a man humming a tune as he read a magazine, and asked, "What are you doing here?" and the man stood up and smiled and said, "I am optimizing my health."

Each person was doing the exact same action in both stories, yet each person had a different perception of what they were doing. Your perceptions and approaches to your health will be the difference maker in what kind of quality of life you have.

This story is about chiropractic but it can be applied in many areas of life. Why are you forgoing dessert tonight or the second helping of dinner? Why did you go to the gym today? Did you force yourself to do 10 minutes of cardio and not just lift weights? Did you add a few new exercises or 5% more weight on your lifts this week?

You had three reasons as well. You could have been lazy and relaxed on your couch eating two bowls of ice cream. Option two is you are trying to create a habit or just know doing the action is better than the alternative, getting fat and unhealthy blood work results at your next doctor visit. Last option is the person who is already in a good routine but wants even more gains and pushes themselves to achieve more with the time they have. Many of us fluctuate between all three motivations throughout the month but your perception of how you feel when doing it is important (sometimes you just plain hate it). More commonly, it's the after effects we love and not always the process: our body looks great, self-esteem improves, blood work is great, disease is 'magically' improving and the list could go on.

Remember, it's only a matter of perception.

12 DOC, DO WHAT YOU DID LAST TIME

I had a conversation with a patient the other day that I thought you might find interesting. The patient was a male in his late 40's. He became a patient because he has chronic low back pain. The first 7 chiropractic adjustments I gave him didn't provide much relief. In fact, in each of those first 7 visits the patient stated that he wasn't feeling any better and wasn't sure if the adjustments were working. When he came in for his 8th chiropractic adjustment, he seemed like he was in a great mood.

I asked him how his body was functioning and he said, "Doc, I feel great! Do whatever you did the last time I was here. That really seemed to work." The thing is the adjustments that I gave this patient were essentially the same every time. So why did he think that the first 7 adjustments weren't doing any good and the 8th adjustment was the one that made all the difference? Because he doesn't understand how the body heals.

The patient gave the 8th adjustment all the credit, but the truth is it was ALL of the adjustments together that made the difference. That is because healing is a process that takes time. If you don't give your body enough time or enough adjustments to heal, it won't heal. You see, each chiropractic adjustment you receive builds on the previous one. Even if you don't feel any better after the first few adjustments, that doesn't mean your body isn't healing, because it is.

Just like it takes years to reposition teeth with braces, it takes several chiropractic adjustments to restore proper movement and alignment with the spine. Make sure you give yourself enough time to heal and get results with your chiropractic care.

Patients become frustrated sometimes because they want to feel better immediately and if they don't get better overnight, they don't think the adjustments are working. If you cut your finger, does the wound heal in 24 hours? No, it takes days before the cut has healed.

When on a diet, do you reach your goal in one week? How about one month? For most of us, absolutely not. In fact, because losing weight takes so much time, and being on our best behavior with food choices every day and every meal, we tend to give up. Same holds true for the gym. Some people want to increase their bench press by 50 pounds but only want to go to the gym twice a week. Guess what? If you put in the time and effort it takes week after week then yes, one day you will accomplish that goal. But it wasn't the 84th visit to the gym or the 45th meal that suddenly caused you to be victorious. Generally, it takes a slow, methodical, consistent effort to do the things in life that are most important.

So to wrap this up, here are three points that I want you to take away from this story:

** Each chiropractic adjustment, meal, visit to the gym you receive builds upon the previous.

** Healing and body changes are processes that take time.

** Chiropractic, diet and exercise work if you give yourself enough time and enough consistency.

What else can you think of that takes time to get results? Can you get a college degree in one year? Can you knit a scarf in one hour? Have you ever tried to write a book...how long did that take? What about being competent at a sport like basketball or running. Each hour of practice builds on the previous and you get good at whatever you desire over time.

13 STUDY SHOWS HOW TO GET MORE OUT OF CHIROPRACTIC

The scientific research periodical, the Journal of Manipulative and Physiological Therapeutics, published a study that will help you... Keep Your Aches, Pains and Stress A Distant Memory

The study divided subjects into two groups. The first group received 12 chiropractic adjustments in one month, followed by a reduced schedule of one adjustment every three weeks for 9 months. The second group only received one month of chiropractic care. The two groups were then compared and evaluated for pain and disability.

Here's What They Found...

The results showed that both groups had similar reductions in pain and disability after the initial 30 days of chiropractic care. However, the big difference was that the group that received one adjustment every three weeks for nine months was able to maintain their reduction in disability. The group that only received one month of care returned to the same levels of disability they were experiencing prior to the initial chiropractic care.

How This Benefits You

Understanding this information could make a big difference for you. More than anything, this study confirms the importance and necessity of taking your spinal health seriously and actually taking care of your back on a regular basis. You know what else needs cleaning on a regular basis? Your teeth! Brush twice daily, floss, use mouth wash, and have your teeth cleaned every 6 months. Here's a **health hack** you may never heard of. Many studies have found that a certain percentage of people who died of a heart attack (a silent killer, meaning you never know if and when you will get one) and others who started having some fever, joint pains etc a few days after having a dental procedure (even just a routine cleaning) saw a certain bacteria in the heart valve tissue that should only be found in the mouth. They theorize that bloody gums transferred the bacteria into the blood stream and somehow settled into the heart. Over time, the bacteria can lead to your death, but you should really experience symptoms and get appropriate treatment way before that. This is why doctors ask if you have had a dental procedure lately. Also, this is one reason why they give you a round of antibiotics before major dental procedures, to kill the bacteria before it can infect you in other areas. My mom always told me to take good care of my teeth and now this study sure gives me an even graver warning to keep my mouth and gums healthy. How about you?

Great health and a wonderful quality of life are created by taking care of your body in all areas on a regular basis. This includes your spine, your teeth, cardiovascular system and so on. If you never use the services out there to improve your health then they obviously can't help much. But if you make it part of the regular activities you do to keep yourself healthy, you will start to experience the benefits that my family and thousands of others experience.

14 WORK INJURY RECOVERY AND WITH FEWER SURGERY: SIGN ME UP

There have been many popular research studies the last few years that prove how effective chiropractic care is. Here is another one!

A study published in the April 2011 issue of the Journal of Occupational and Environmental Medicine suggests that when it comes to work-related low back pain, the risk of disability recurrence is lower for patients treated primarily by a chiropractic doctor compared to patients treated by a physical therapist or a medical physician. So not only were the patients who received chiropractic care instead of medical care having less recurrence of back pain, they were also spending less money.

This study is more good news for chiropractic patients. Another study looked at a group of people who all met the criteria for low back surgery. Half went to surgery and the other half did chiropractic. In the chiropractic group, 60% saw improvement and didn't need surgery after all, and the other 40% who had the surgery had better outcomes than those who didn't have chiropractic to start with. I personally still like the statistics that shows about an 85% success rate in general with chiropractics but for those who have never got an adjustment and qualify for surgery, maybe it's time to give it a try.

About nine studies evaluated the cost, drug use, long-term disability and a few other parameters after a work-related accident. They looked at physical therapy, medical care and chiropractic care to see how each played out. I won't bore you with all the specifics but they found that chiropractic care reduced all the important parameters on average 17.25% better than physical therapy and 100.25% better when compared to medical care. Am I claiming superiority? No way. In my opinion, it is just proving the case that chiropractic should be included in standards of care. Not only should it be included but it should be one of the first referrals given in my opinion, assuming no fractures, concussions or other serious life threatening issues. It cuts cost because we do fewer units of billable exercise than physical therapy and it never has the high cost of surgery. Depending on the case, like following knee and shoulder surgeries, a patient will typically find that physical therapy is more specialized to treat these recoveries.

Remember, this is a discussion of work-related injuries, but you can transfer some of these results to "weekend warrior" sports injuries, and other "I hurt myself doing XYZ activity" as well. So as you can see, there's lots of great information coming out that is proving what we already knew, that chiropractic care is one of the safest, most affordable and best treatments for back pain.

The bottom line is that chiropractic care just works. It helps people with pain, it helps athletes perform better, it helps children through their growth and development and it helps people's overall quality of life.

15 BLUEPRINT TO REBOOT YOUR NERVOUS SYSTEM: CHIROPRACTIC SUMMARY

When I ask patients what the most important system of the body is, they tend to say "blood and heart." I can understand why they would think that. With all the commercials on TV talking about lowering cholesterol, high blood pressure, heart attack prevention and the most common lab tests run by doctors, they all deal with stuff floating in your blood. Who can blame them for getting the wrong answer. Truth be told, the nervous system is actually numero uno.

The nervous system is the master coordinator and controller of all your body's organs and structures. Without a nerve impulse traveling throughout your body, it would cease to function. My youngest brother was paralyzed from the waist down. Did his legs still grow, yes. Did his skin heal after being cut, yes. Was his brain functioning normally and could he learn like people who could walk, yes. What was the problem then? The area of his spinal cord that involuntarily transmits pain, temperature, vibration, and contracting muscles were permanently damaged only in the location that connected his legs. I know we have all heard stories of someone breaking their neck and becoming paralyzed from the neck down. In fact, these people may not even be able to breathe anymore without a machine because the nerve impulse stops at the neck due to the damage and anything downstream (lungs, arms, legs) will no longer work. The blood is pumping and keeping the organs alive with oxygen, but movement is no longer possible. Obviously, you need both blood and nerves to survive. If blood gets cut off to a finger for a long enough time, the finger turns black and can literally fall off. That's scary too. If your heart stops beating, you die. The body is much like a car. If the engine is running but the transmission is broken or a tire is missing, good luck going anywhere. If the heart or lungs or nerves stop working, your body will either die or cease to function as intended.

What do you do to maintain the health of your nervous system? Did you know that there is even a way to maintain it? I mean, we brush our teeth every day so we can prevent cavities because the damage of neglect is obvious. We even wear sunscreen on our face because our skin will wrinkle and, if we aren't careful, cancer can form. Damage to our nervous system can occur because of direct trauma, like a car accident, but more commonly, slow wear and tear is the culprit. Our vertebrae are the armor to protect our spinal cord. The spinal cord is inside a cavity that runs vertically through the entire spine. Nerves branch off the spinal cord and travel down to the arm, the chest, and the legs. Each vertebra has two openings that these nerves must pass through before going to its appropriate area. Neglecting our spine (vertebrae) over time will lead to arthritis and degeneration. Generally this manifests as extra bone growth (spurs) at the front of the vertebrae, but more importantly, these spurs can form at the exit point of nerves and cause damage. The spurs are sharp and can cut and irritate the muscles, ligaments and nerves in that area. Think of a rope rubbing against a pair of scissors all day long; the scissors make contact with the rope and will fray it. These spurs can cause swelling, pressure and pain. Disc bulges and herniations are also issues that can cause problems to these nerves and even the spinal cord. Symptoms of numbness, pain, muscle tightness, shooting electric sensations and tingling are all signs of nerve damage. Have you ever hit your "funny bone?" Well, that sharp shooting pain that goes to your fingers is actually the nerve letting you know that you smashed it. Can you imagine having that feeling for days, weeks or months like some of my patients do?

Arthritis of the spine is a slow process and will generally exhibit no signs or warnings for a long time. Chiropractors call this slowly forming process of arthritis that causes the nervous system to malfunction a subluxation. But this is not entirely appropriate as, medically speaking, a subluxation means a joint that is almost dislocated. Obviously a chiropractor doesn't try to put back (adjust) an almost dislocated vertebrae. What they are referring to is when a pair of vertebrae is stuck in a position and unable to move freely like they are supposed to. Sometimes it is obvious if you can't straighten your neck after falling asleep all night on your sofa's armrest. Other times, if you are trained to watch somebody bend over or walk and evaluate their motions, you will see that a person is compensating somewhere. Maybe when they walk, they raise their hip higher on one side than the other, and upon questioning them, they say, "Yes, this side hurts but if I walk like this the pain goes away." Oftentimes, it's a slow progression and they don't even recognize an issue until someone points it out.

A doctor of chiropractic (8 years of school) is trained to find these misalignments, where vertebrae are stuck, and correct them. Why correct them? Research has shown over and over again that a joint that doesn't move freely develops arthritis: knees, elbows and, yes, the spine. In fact, some studies of spine and joint arthritis in pigs will immobilize a certain joint and then inject that joint with a special chemical that will cause rapid onset of degeneration. Then they deliver adjustments to that joint and study what happens to the nerves and surrounding tissues. Research has found reduced inflammation and pain signals and increased motion following joint adjustment.

One point I may have glossed over is that this progression is typically painless. Pain is a very helpful signal to our body. When we step on a piece of glass, it hurts. If we didn't have this warning, we could do some serious damage by walking on glass all day. If we didn't have pain, how would we know that the shower temperature was too hot and would burn us? However, subluxations (an unfamiliar topic to most people) are not the only things that have consequences that start out painlessly. Diabetes, high blood pressure, high cholesterol and high triglycerides all have a painless progression. Scarfing down donuts, French bread and cheese our entire life coupled with not exercising finally catches up to us in our 30s or 40s. We go to the doctor's office for a routine check-up and get some blood work done. The doctor looks straight into our eyes and informs us that all these markers are high saying, "I will give you 3 months to show some progress of lowering them, or you will be on these 4 drugs for the rest of your life. If you choose to continue to eat like you do, we will max out the dose."

By not controlling your conditions, you may lose your vision, your kidneys will fail, you may suffer a heart attack or a stroke might paralyze half your body causing you to be a burden on your family, or you might just die right there on the spot (which at one point in time for 50% of the people, the first warning sign that someone had a blood/heart issue was the heart attack). Luckily, a misaligned vertebrae, subluxation, isn't going to kill while you shop at the mall. Heck, most people have never even gone to a chiropractor. Does that mean they shouldn't go and shouldn't take care of their nervous system though? I don't think so. We brush our teeth at home and for some people that is still not enough to prevent cavities from slowly and painlessly forming. Once the tooth hurts, the dentist fixes it.

Volumes of research have been published in peer reviewed journals over the past 30 years proving over and over again how adjusting the spine has helped people get rid of low back and neck pain, not to mention the cost savings. They have covered different adjusting techniques, conditions the patient might experience, how degeneration occurs, biomechanical studies, comparing adjustments to injections, whether muscle massage and exercise is necessary or not and the list goes on and on. Studies have been done that show how this saves insurance companies and governments money by having chiropractors on the plans and how people were able to get back to work quicker and avoid long-term disabilities compared to groups that didn't utilize a doctor of chiropractic. Personally, I don't really care if professional athletes use something but many of them do utilize chiropractic adjustment and offer credit to the adjustment as a way for them to not only recover faster, but to give them the edge. This makes sense because flexibility increases, reaction times improve and many other attributes that are worthy of an athlete's time have a positive impact.

The takeaway secret is this. Remove the subluxations from your spine. Keep your spine healthy and stop the progression of arthritis from occurring in the first place. If you are already in pain, have a limited range of motion or you just know something isn't quite right in a joint of yours, maybe it is time to visit a chiropractor. Headaches might be common but they sure aren't normal and you don't have to live with them. Numbness and tingling in your hands, arm, legs or feet are also not normal and the longer you wait the worse it will get. Much like it's better to fix a cavity when it's small so you don't need a root canal, it's easier to correct a spine issue when it's fresh rather than waiting till you're bent over in pain for months. Furthermore, you can't fix your own tooth cavities and you can't fix your own spine. I know some of you are scared of the cracking sound and being twisted. That's ok, you can ask or find someone who uses an adjusting instrument. These instruments are gentle, require no twisting or popping, and research has shown that they are just as effective as the more standard manual adjustment. Where can you go to find one? Ask your social media friends who they go to. If you are uncomfortable with the doctor's personality, financial options, staff or whatever during the consultation, just excuse yourself and find a different one. Everybody practices a little differently and we each have our own personality and those may not gel with you. Don't give up on improving your health through proper nerve integrity. Try it for a month or two and I am confident you will notice a difference.

16 THE 5 ESSENTIAL HABITS OF GREAT HEALTH + 6 BONUSES

Today I want to share with you five habits the healthiest people in the world have that makes them super healthy. The easiest way to achieve success in anything is to COPY the people who are already successful at it. The hardest part of being successful is not only knowing what to do, but also taking action and doing it. Learn what the healthiest people in the world do and then take action!

Let's get started with the 5 Essential Habits of Great Health.

```
================================
```
Habit #1: The Habit of Adequate Rest
```
================================
```

You've got to get your sleep if you expect to be healthy and productive. Think about a rechargeable battery for a second. What happens when a rechargeable battery wears out? You put it back into the charger so it gets its power back. What happens if you don't recharge the batteries when they wear down? They don't work!

Your body is just like a rechargeable battery. You have to RECHARGE your body if you want to be able to perform. Too often we are on overdrive, running ourselves into the ground, under a lot of stress and, to make matters worse, we aren't getting enough sleep to keep up. If you don't give your body enough rest and time to recharge, your body will start to wear down. Once your body wears down, it doesn't work correctly. You won't be as productive in any area of your life and you could even end up getting sick. Have you experienced a lack of energy around noon, brain fog, disorientation and irritability the day following a 2 a.m. bedtime? Another example of lack of adequate sleep would be the jet lag feeling after a long flight.

So how much sleep should we get each night? Studies say 7 to 8 hours a night. If you are getting less than that, even if you are feeling pretty good, your body is SLOWLY wearing out. Have trouble sleeping? Many of my patients report that getting chiropractic care helps them sleep better. Exercising on a regular basis also helps.

Your goal: Try to get at least 7-8 hours of sleep each night.

================================
Habit #2: The Habit of Healthy Eating
================================

I think we all know that it's important to eat well. Think of food as fuel. When you go to the gas station, you usually have the following fuel choices: 85, 87, and 91. What if your choices instead looked like this: 40, 65, 91? Would you fill your tank with the 40 octane? I doubt you would. Your car would run sluggishly.

If you consistently eat foods that are unhealthy for you, just like a low grade of gasoline in your car, your body will run poorly. The better the food you put in your body, the better your body will perform. If you want to perform at a high level at work, with your family and with your hobbies then you need to give your body the proper fuel to make that happen.

Your goal: Eat a little healthier. Here are some suggestions:

1. Drink pure water. Get a really good water filter or buy purified water. Take your body weight and divide by two and drink that many ounces of water each day.
2. Supplement your diet with omega-3 fish oil, preferably EPA/DHA, with about 1000mg of these two ingredients. Many bottles have 1000mg but only 500mg total of EPA/DHA, but you need 1000mg.
3. Shop the outer aisles of the grocery store. That's where all of the "live" foods are; fruits, vegetables, fish, meats, and poultry. Avoid processed foods.
4. Have your sinful desires, but have them in moderation. Often it's the portions we eat that are the problem. Adopt the 80/20 rule. Eat really well 80% of the time and blow it for 20%.
5. Avoid artificial sweeteners. I tackle this topic later in the book. Suffice it to say, some people are sensitive to the chemicals, some people feel it may cause cancer and others say its fine because the government says it is.
6. Do not eat foods with "trans fats". The label will say partially hydrogenated oil. Trans fats are very bad for you. Many food manufacturers are not cooking with this type of oil anymore, but make sure you read the label.
7. Cut your portions down. Eat a little less at each sitting. I personally lost 11 pounds in 7 weeks by cutting my portions down and exercising. I did it and so can you.

Two Simple Changes to Your Plate that Fool Your Hunger Meter

Part 1: Seems to me that our plates, bowls and cups just keep getting bigger and bigger over the years. It also takes a bigger spoonful of casserole and larger chicken breasts to fill that plate. For some reason, we have this need to fill up the whole plate and only then will we "feel full" from our meal. That means a lot more calories. Psychologically, we want those plates full of food and if you ever just put ½ a spoonful of vegetables and everything else, you look at your plate and think, "what am I, a 7 year old?" As a side note, if you really want to lose weight, focus 90% of your energy on controlling your food intake. Exercise has many benefits (heart and lung function improve, circulation is better, sleep improves, natural anti-depressant, etc.) but those 200 calories burned with a ½ hour run will never offset the bottle of beer and two scoops of ice cream over dinner.

The secret is to start using smaller plates and bowls. I'm no expert, but plate sizes come in large, medium and ones for your coffee/tea cup. I recommend using the medium size "salad or bread" plate. If you eat a plate full of food, even if it is a smaller plate, psychologically, we suddenly feel satisfied. Let's outsmart our own brains and counterproductive habits by reducing our plate size. Smaller plates combined with no second servings could easily mean you cut 20-30% off your calories for that meal. Even more if you are someone who eats more than one meal a day, like it's a Las Vegas buffet and needs to fill that uncomfortable belly bulge, unbutton my pants "ahh, pressure relief", like I just ate a Thanksgiving dinner feeling. You might be so used to stuffing your belly that it has grown much bigger than normal and you are nervous that, if you eat smaller portions, you will not get that full sensation and be uncomfortably hungry all day long. If this describes your concern, then have no fear, I cover this issue later in this book.

Let's get back to talking plate size, shall we? Grab that smaller plate and serve one spoonful of mashed potatoes, carrots, eggplant and ½ a chicken breast and your plate is overflowing all of a sudden. Admit it, when you take that last bite ,it's hard to say you haven't eaten a ton of food. Same goes with your bowls and cups. A dainty tea cup full of ice cream is going to be way less calories than an 18 oz coffee mug. Remember when we were kids and the cafeteria at school gave us that little bitty carton of ice cream with a wooden spoon? That size is about ½ a cup and that, my friends, is the 120-180 calories per serving written on the grown-up size cartons of ice cream. I hate to break it to you, but a pint of ice cream is still 4 servings. Take your time and enjoy each bite. How many times have you eaten a delicious cookie, like a macadamia nut-cranberry sugar cookie, and suddenly realized how fast you devoured it and grab a second. Slow down and really savor it. That was a 300 calorie mistake, or 1 hour of running to offset it. Later I give you another hack on how to be mindful and slow down so that you can enjoy all food, especially snacks.

Part 2: The second part of this hack is contrasting plate colors. I saw a documentary on TV and they did an experiment where customers ate a bowl of soup, but the bowl had a device rigged to it that would allow the soup to continue to replenish without the eater knowing. The point was to see how much someone would consume before stopping due to feeling full, because they would never "finish the bowl" and have the satisfaction of an empty bottom. The results were staggering:

more was consumed when the bowls were the same colors as the soup. When the bowl was a contrasting color to the soup, they were able to stop themselves much sooner, maybe 20-30% sooner. So if you have the habit of eating a whole bunch of tomato-based red food, then you might benefit from white or black plates instead of those cool red ones you love. Imagine eating 10 mozzarella cheese sticks for a whopping 800 calories. Now if you cut out 30%, you only eat 7 sticks of cheese for 560 calories and saved yourself an hour of exercise in the long run to burn off those extra 240 calories. You might be saying to yourself, seven cheese sticks is just gross and excessive, I would only eat 4 max. Get off your high horse because I bet you can eat up two bowls of chips and salsa at the local Mexican joint or a hefty slice of blueberry cobbler cheesecake smothered in ice cream after a 12 oz rib-eye and gigantic baked potato.

Lesson Learned Living in China

I learned a few tricks for cooking. Ginger and spicy pepper-flake oil are secret ingredients to make a normal dish become fresh and extraordinary.

Why do the Chinese cut their food so small? The reason they cut their meat and vegetables so small and thin is because they use chopsticks and, as an extra bonus, everything cooks quicker. It's too hard to pick up a 12oz ribeye steak with chopsticks and chew on it like a caveman. Am I advocating you switch to chopsticks, no. However, you can still adopt some of the principles to better serve your waist line. If you chop up a chicken breast into bite size pieces and then cook it, that one breast will be so scattered throughout your dish that it can feed 2 or 3 people. Pair it with chopped veggies and not only does everything cook faster, but the spices and flavor penetrate more of your food's surface area. Now every bite is bursting with goodness. Now you can combine the chicken and vegetables (assuming you matched spices) and have a nice chopped dish you can take a spoonful or two of for lunch.

My parents told us after we were adults, spaghetti was a great meal because pasta is cheap and one pound of ground beef cut small and spread out in a sauce goes a long way to feeding a family of five. I have to remind my wife sometimes when we are plating our meal: Sweet Love of Mine, all we cooked was an organic chicken breast (smaller than the frozen big box store breasts), ½ a carrot, (onions, bell peppers and garlic do not count to me as a dish-they're used for flavor) and 1 potato (or ½ an eggplant or 6 bok choy all substituted for the potato)... we can eat everything, no need for leftovers. Seriously though, it's chopped into bite size portions and it looks and feels like you are eating a ton. I dare you to try it.

Secret Chinese Pepper Flake Oil Recipe:

Get some fresh red pepper flakes. They are what come in packets to sprinkle on pizza. Put a ½ cup into a small ceramic or porcelain bowl that has a detachable lid. The pepper flakes need to be very slightly moist, not soaking wet and definitely no standing water. Next, heat up some peanut oil, sunflower oil or another high cooking temperature oil. You don't want to use extra virgin olive oil because the oil burns at too low of a temperature and I wouldn't recommend coconut oil unless you just like everything tasting tropical. Heat the oil until it is super hot but not burnt and take the lid off the ceramic bowl with the flakes in. You will be pouring a little bit of the oil on top of the flakes and it will sizzle and pop so you might want a helper to use the lid as a shield from the oil popping and hitting your hand or clothes. Once you pour a little oil on top of the flakes, it will bubble up and when it calms down a little then use a spoon to stir the flakes. Then pour more oil and stir and repeat until it seems like all the flakes are saturated with oil. If you see any dry flakes, put more hot oil on it. This method cooks (and incinerates some) of the pepper flakes. To use, just put a teaspoon at a time in your soups, or mix some into your veggies or meat while you cook. Yes, it is spicy (and oily) so add slowly.

When It's Food Time, Don't Sit In Front of Electronics

A study followed freshman girls for one semester and found that those who ate in front of the TV or while on a phone gained 15 pounds compared to those who did not. That is a ton of weight to try and burn off. Moral of the story, when it is time to eat, just eat and talk, don't be distracted by electronic gadgets.

BE MINDFUL OF WHEN AND HOW YOU EAT

A study showed that being conscious, aware and mindful of your eating helps you stay thin. This means taking your time to eat. It can take your stomach 30 minutes to tell the brain, "Hey, I'm stuffed-go ahead and shut off the 'I'm still Hungry' chemicals." The study also showed that overweight people tend to only chew their food 15 times before swallowing... aka, it was shoveled down. Thin people chewed their food an average of 45 times. Have you ever chewed anything that long? It's hard to do.

Action step: Aim for 45 but be happy and feel accomplished when starting out at 25 chews before you swallow. "I don't want to count, how boring, and besides I'm busy socializing," I can hear you complain. Ok, go buy a step clicker (some airline flight attendants can be seen with a little metal box with a trigger they click as they count the passengers before take-off) and click every time you chew, then look at it before swallowing. You should notice that you are able to savor all the delicious flavors from each bite of food. I've caught myself chewing a piece of lamb, swallowing while it's still chunky only to quickly grab another piece. Typically, it's on that second piece where I notice I'm not even enjoying the bite in my mouth and already looking to eat more. Slow down Justin, chew it more and savor all the flavors from each bite. Maybe this is less exciting for broccoli but it comes in handy when limiting yourself to a single cookie. Remember, no single item of food is bad or evil and neither are you for eating it, so don't feel any guilt or shame for it.

==================================
Habit #3: The Habit of Regular Exercise
==================================

Again, we all know that exercise is important. I know that you know it would be extremely beneficial if you exercised on a regular basis. If we all know that exercise is such a great thing to do, then the million dollar question is, why don't we do it? Are we really too busy to take care of ourselves? Some say yes, but that's not the correct answer.

Saying you are too busy to keep yourself healthy is like saying you are too busy driving on the highway to pull over for gas. If you are driving on the highway, at some point you will have to pull over for gas if you want to keep driving - do you agree?

Well, if you are "too busy" to put yourself first once in a while, guess what? You are going to burn out and your fast-paced lifestyle will get the better of you. Getting regular exercise is VITALLY important to your health in so many ways.

When we don't exercise regularly, here's what we are doing to ourselves:

- We increase our chance of heart disease
- We shorten our life span
- We increase our chances of depression and anxiety
- We don't sleep as well
- We don't have as much energy
- We gain weight
- We lose our normal flexibility and become stiffer

Who wants all those bad things in their life? I know you don't want that. I know I don't. If you don't take time for your health, you'll have to make time for your sickness. Read that again and let it soak in. There are just too many positive benefits from keeping yourself active and exercising that there is really no good excuse not to.

Your goal: Rearrange your priorities and time to include some form of exercise on a regular basis.

Start slow, and try to build up to at least 30 minutes 4-5 times a week. You don't have to spend a lot of money and you don't have to join a gym if you don't want to. Just get out and take a brisk walk every day and it will do wonders for your health.

Two Tidbits about Consistency and Long-Term Goals

Each chiropractic adjustment, meal, or visit to the gym you receive builds upon the previous. The main difference between someone who has lost 20 pounds on a specific diet versus 5 pounds is the 20 pounds person stuck with it 3-4 times as long. You just can't rush results. If I want to increase my bicep size by 3 inches, I can either strap a ballon to my arm or I can go to the gym for 9 months and gain the muscle. Every bicep curl, push up, protein shake and pull up over the weeks is required for these long term goals to be actualized. Chiropractic, diet, and exercise works if you give yourself enough time and enough consistency.

====================
Habit #4: A Good Attitude
====================

You've got to have a good attitude if you expect to have great health. I have never seen someone with a lousy attitude have great health. How you think and how you act has tremendous power.

Here's what you don't want:

- To be negative about everything
- To be a constant complainer
- To constantly criticize others
- To blame others
- To be a victim

Here's what you do want:

- Be complimentary to people
- Take 100% responsibility for your health and your life
- Have a positive outlook on life
- Do not blame others
- Put a smile on your face. Be happy!

Your Goal: Identify areas of your attitude that could be improved and work on them. Life is just too short to be negative.

Habit #5:
Healthy and Proper Function of Your Central Nervous System

For your body to be healthy, your nervous system must be working properly. Your nervous system is made up of your brain, spinal cord and all the nerves in your body. If there's any interference with your nervous system, it's literally impossible for you to have optimal health. Your brain communicates with the rest of your body by sending messages through the nerve to every cell, tissue, organ and system in the body.

What happens if you have a subluxation (vertebrae that are misaligned or not moving properly)? The subluxation causes interference to the nervous system. This causes your body to malfunction. That's why it's so important that you don't have subluxations in your spine causing interference in your nervous system. Chiropractic adjustments are the best treatment in the world to keep the spine and nervous system healthy.

Many people new to chiropractic think adjustments are just for pain, but the truth is, chiropractic care is designed to improve the function and performance of your entire body. Just ask all the professional athletes who use chiropractic care on a regular basis to improve their performance!

That's why great spinal health is so important to having great overall health. If you want to know what I do, I get adjusted every 3 to 6 weeks. My wife does too. And if I had kids, they would be adjusted once a month as well.

Your goal: Make your spinal health a bigger priority in your life. Get adjustments on a 4-12 week basis to keep your nervous system working at an optimal level.

17 THE TRUTH ABOUT FAT IN YOUR DIET

I found some very interesting information on "fat" in our diet that I wanted to share with you. The question is..."Do we have too much fat in our diets?" The answer may surprise you. Any way you look at it, there's a debate over whether or not America's health problems are a consequence of a "high fat" diet.

Here's the deal: Americans are not eating a diet abnormally high in fat. Before this idea became commercialized, politicized, used to market and sell products, distorted by vegetarian wishes and adopted by the "mass media", no one ever really proved that our diets are too high in fat. The average American intakes 35% of their calories from fat. Seem like a lot? Look closer.

Surviving native pre-agrarian (pre-agricultural diet) cultures average 38% of their calories from fat. It's not uncommon for them to have 50% of their caloric intake come from fat and even with this fat intake, they do not suffer from the epidemic heart disease problem afflicting America. That is our prototypical diet. We've eaten this way for millions of years. Now, don't get me wrong, there are definite problems with modern dietary fat but lowering your fat intake will only worsen your deviation from your natural diet.

So what should we do? In today's diet, we typically eat too many carbohydrates. So try to lower your total carbs and stay away from carbohydrates that have a high glycemic index. Some foods that have a high glycemic index are cereals, potatoes, breads and pastas. Fat is not necessarily the enemy. You do not want to give up having fat in your diet. The key is to choose "healthy fats" and monitor your carbohydrates.

18 NEW CONCEPT: KETOGENIC BASED DIETS

This book is not the place to fully explore ketogenic or modified ketosis diets. The 30,000 foot view is that you eat 5-15% carbs, 20-30% protein and the rest is fat. Not just any fat will do though. The proponents of this lifestyle of eating in a nutshell recommend coconut oils, medium chain triglycerides (the 8 and 10 branch version with the 8 being the best available), exogenous ketones, high fat veggies like avocados and nuts, and dairy products (but some are against too much dairy because of the carb component). Many people who experiment with this diet end up losing a lot of weight because they accidentally over-restrict calories. It's surprisingly hard to eat 70% of your diet as fat. You can't just eat 5 steaks a day either, because excessive protein intake also breaks down and can be used like a carb instead of like a fat. You may have heard of people drinking coffee with MCT oil (95% 8 chain) and grass fed butter and how it keeps them full and mentally alert. The amount of fat consumed causes your satiety to last throughout the morning and many claim they feel their brain is working on all cylinders.

A ketosis diet has been proven to help with epilepsy seizures which diminish for those whom standard medicine just doesn't work, especially children. Also, whether someone is sticking to a pure ketosis based diet or getting help with exogenous ketones, there are studies showing positive effects with reducing certain cancers, prolonging life if diagnosed with certain brain cancers, and reducing the side effects of chemotherapy, celiac and Crohn's Disease.

Research it online for yourself. There are some really good podcast episodes out there that go into lots of detail on this topic. I'm not an expert on it, but I wanted to bring it to your attention. I firmly believe that it's a shame the low carb gurus lost the battle to the low fat gurus decades ago. You can already see the buzz that margarine is bad and butter is good again, egg yolks aren't killing you, and more often you will hear about reducing your sugar intake than in years past.

Extra Tidbit: Sugar Creates Inflammation

Excessive amounts of sugar in our diet, 45-60% carbohydrates (think of those who drink lots of soda, alcohol, breads, desserts, i.e. a typical Western Society Diet) create inflammation in the body, burn out our pancreas and lead to diabetes. All this has serious consequences like loss of eyesight, amputated feet and kidney failure. The sugar molecule circulates in our blood and arteries. The sugar molecule looks like a spikey ball and when a surplus is running through the arteries, it has a tendency to scrape and cut the interior artery wall along the way. Regardless if you get a scrape on your skin, the artery going to your lung, leg, or kidney, the results are the same; inflammation occurs and that creates a little swelling, the tissue is sensitive and the scrapes have caused some injury. The next step involves the fat we have been eating that accompanies a lot of sugary products. Fat, which is sticky, floats around inside the artery and starts to fill into these cuts. Over time, this causes artery plaque to build up and clogs the arteries. A standard approach to fix the problem is to just limit the fat floating around. I'm sorry but that's just like continuingly adding air to your car tire that has a screw poking through it. Remove the screw, patch the tire and you can stop adding air to it every other day. In our artery health, remove the excessive amounts of sugar causing the cuts and inflammation to begin with and the fat will just float on by. The caveat is that you need to be eating healthy fats. The way ketosis diets work is that your body can switch from using predominantly sugar-based energy to a more calorie rich fat energy base. If you decide to start chowing down on a bunch of fat but you don't limit that carb intake, then you will notice that your waist line will increase and your blood work will also look dismal. Ketosis based eating requires that really low carb intake to work correctly, so consider this your warning.

Last side note: I also think that there is a link to high carb intake and all the fibromyalgia, gluten intolerance, sluggish feeling and brain fog so many of us live with. Give yourself a 60 day gluten free eating challenge and see how you feel. Seriously, don't cheat during these 60 days because the gluten molecule can linger around for almost two weeks, secretly sabotaging your efforts. I say secretly because real gluten intolerant people can have near immediate diarrhea and migraines if they ingest gluten. They can continue to feel icky for a few days while the body readjusts. I have a hard time believing that so many people are truly gluten intolerant (celiac disease), but I wouldn't be surprised if many, at a minimum, are somewhat sensitive to the amounts they ingest and could see an overall health benefit by removing those inflaming carbs and gluten.

Word of Caution: Why Am I so Grumpy When Off the Carbs?

If you ever tried to cut carbs out for a day, you will remember feeling grumpy, irritable, may be depressed with some serious cravings for sugar. It's a highly addictive substance but if you reduce the intake for a week or so, your body adapts and doesn't crave it as much. Remember that no food is evil, no food is truly bad for you (in low amounts) and you shouldn't feel guilty or shameful if you eat something. We all know donuts have no reason to ever be in our mouth, but when you do eat it, just eat one (not 3), and don't feel guilty about that one indulgence. Just enjoy it since you already chose to eat it. Many people comment that after getting off the junk for a few weeks, the same foods they used to enjoy are no longer enjoyable. We all have our kryptonite so just indulge sparingly and wisely.

Secret Hack: Don't Let Fake Sugar Fake You Out

Avoid artificial sweeteners and soda of all types. It is pure empty calories and the 'diet' ones have artificial sweeteners that may or may not have long-term direct or indirect negative effects on our bodies. I read that those who drink diet soda are typically fatter because the part of our brain that says, "AHH sugar" is never activated so we eat desserts. Look, I'll play devil's advocate with you. I won't give up soda but I also don't want diabetes and the extra weight. Ok, maybe drink the artificial sweeteners and see what happens long term. To lessen the risk, just drink one 12 ounce can a day or, if you can handle it, only drink 2-3 a week. Switching to coffee or tea is another option. If your diet is low in carbs and sugars and you drink diet beverages, then you might not get diabetes and that's a good thing. Research is conflicting on how bad, or cancer causing, the artificial sweeteners are anyway.

However, here are some more disturbing thoughts about artificial sweeteners for women. Those who drink two or more sodas per day have a 30% higher chance of a cardiovascular event. Here's one last piece of summarized research that I read at some point that stuck with me. Researchers looked at the bacteria in the gut of artificial sweetener consuming mice and it was not only different than those who just ate normal sugar, but it led to higher blood sugar levels. This is the opposite of what you would assume because we are supposed to be consuming fake sugar to avoid high blood sugar levels. If that isn't weird enough, if they transferred the feces of artificial sweetener mice into the sugar consumers, those rats quickly started having high blood sugar levels when they were normal before. I don't remember all the details about how much artificial sweetener they ate, and the other finer details, but I remember reading it and thinking, well I better cut way back on the fake stuff and just limit my intake of desserts and bread anyway.

Bonus Tip about Sugar Alcohols:

Have you heard of sugar alcohols (they are not "get drunk" alcohols)? There is a chewing gum that uses xylitol as a sweetener. Not only are the calories negligible, but teeth bacteria can't use it for food so your mouth can actually be healthier. Sugar alcohols in general are about 70% as sweet as sugar but xylitol can cause diarrhea if consumed in excessive amounts. Everybody responds differently but if you are only consuming 2-4 teaspoons a day, you should be ok. Another version of sugar alcohol that may cause some dehydration or reflux but not diarrhea is erythritol. It has the same properties but has a slight cooling sensation in high amounts so if you bake with it you do need to use real sugar to counteract it. With that said, erythritol is my go-to because it has even fewer calories than xylitol, it does not raise blood sugar levels, has better dental cavity prevention, and the gut has a significantly less chance of diarrhea because of how it is absorbed. Both xylitol and erythritol are actually naturally occurring in fruits and the latter in fermented foods. Go online and you can find articles on Wikipedia as well as How To Cook type sites for more information. Remember that moderation in life is best, and I hope you aren't eating a ton of sugar or alternative sugars each day regardless of what they are. Less is more. Lastly, I prefer erythritol over stevia products. Stevia tends to have an aftertaste and these days companies are modifying it to try and remove that aftertaste. I just wonder if after the modifications it can potentially cause issues long term like your pink, blue and yellow fake sweetener packets.

19 QUICK STEPS TO MASTERING FOOD LABELS

I want to share with you some quick tips on how you can evaluate a food label in 15 seconds or less and know if that food is healthy or not! It's really important to know how to read the basics of a food label because sometimes that's the only way you're going to know what you're really eating. Here's a quick checklist you can use to evaluate the foods you are buying.

====================
Trans and saturated fats
====================

In the U.S., all packaged foods come with a nutrition facts label. The first place my eyes go to is the fat content. I draw my personal line in the sand at trans fats. We don't need it, and there is always another food option without it. Trans fat is man-made fat that comes from dubious preparation processes. If an item has any, it goes back on the shelf.

Next, I look at saturated fat. We don't need much of it, and if we eat meat or dairy products, then we have probably met our requirements without needing it in our other foods. Next to the number of grams, you'll see the percentage of your daily requirement that the food contains, eliminating the need for math. If that number is high, be wary. Of course, you must evaluate what you're buying. Olive oil, for example, is a fat, so it's going to have a high number. However, you don't use much. Potato chips, on the other hand, would have a lower number, but you might eat the entire bag, so you should consider that. But that's obvious stuff, right?

=====
Sugar
=====

Get instantly suspicious if this number is high. Sports foods are supposed to have sugar because you want to quickly replace blood glycogen lost during exercise. All other foods don't need it. If you're buying a dessert item, you'll expect a high ratio of sugar, but for anything else, you're probably getting a cheap product that's poorly produced. Remember that many "low-fat" foods have a lot of sugar--it's not technically fat, it just makes you fat.

Wheat flour, rice flour and other starchy ingredients are at the top of the ingredient list on most frozen foods. You'll find that many have as much as 40 grams of carbohydrate per serving, with only a few grams of fiber. When you see that, this is your clue that you're looking at a high-glycemic food that will spike your blood sugar, promote fat storage and contribute to chronic disease.

Sodium

Prepared foods usually have high levels of sodium. Also, oftentimes, you can find an "organic, non-fat, low-carb," purely healthy sounding food item that has over 1,000 milligrams of sodium, which is around half of your recommended daily allowance (RDA). What you're generally looking for from these three "s" ingredients (saturated fat, sugar and sodium) is a low number, and it only takes a few seconds to figure it out.

Fat, Protein and Carbs Ratio

When choosing a food, you probably already know a few things about it. If it's butter, you'll expect all fat, candy will be high in sugar and things that sit on a shelf may have a lot of sodium. For meals, however, you'll want to take a quick notation of the amount of fat, protein and carbs.

If you're on a strict diet, this ratio is very important, but if you're not, you just want some balance. A nice round number is 30-40 percent carbs, 30 percent protein and 30-40 percent fat. You can then assume that your prepared meals would be better if they reflect a similar balance.

Length of Ingredient List

Now just take a quick glance at where it says "Ingredients". If it's under about 10 items, don't worry about it. If there's a long list of ingredients, take caution. There will be ingredients that you can't even pronounce that you might not want to be eating. If it's somewhere in the middle, I may take a closer look, but in general I keep it simple.

========
Summary
========

There are a few "evil offender" ingredients that people tend to look for, but we've covered them. By checking off the trans-fats, sugar and sodium listed above, we're assured there won't be any MSG, high fructose corn syrup or hydrogenated oils in this section. By adding a mere 15 seconds to look at each item, you may not have the perfect diet, but you can certainly make sure it's not terrible. This is not an exact science, but your diet doesn't have to be either. Eat better and get more exercise. Beyond this, we're nitpicking.

20 BEING HUNGRY AND DEALING WITH IT

Earlier in the book I mentioned that I've lost nearly 30 pounds since my heaviest in 2013. Sure, I fluctuated 10 pounds at times but I am now aware of how it happens and I've learned how to lose it again. Believe me, it's just easier to keep it off and limit my desserts, bread, and cheese than to have to mentally deal with having chubbiness and staying strict on a lower calorie diet.

Have you ever been hungry? I'm serious. Have you ever been so busy that you skip lunch and 7 o'clock comes around and the stomach pain hits you? (I understand for some people they would get a headache if they went that long without a meal and so they not only feel hungry but have a throbbing headache as well, but I can help with that too. For now, let's look at the person who only feels hunger.) Was it really painful or was it more of an uncomfortable sensation? My guess is the latter.

My challenge for you is to embrace that feeling for one day. Purposely skip lunch and be mindful and aware of how your brain and belly feel. Are you grumpy, less productive at work, your stomach gurgles or some other symptom? Stay aware of that feeling around lunch time and just focus on it for 60 minutes before deciding to eat (a smaller portion meal, of course). Did you die from the ache? Nope! Here's my point, having a little hunger sensation is not going to hurt you or really bother you that much. Embrace it and try to sit with that feeling for an extra hour or so. It gets easier if you do it for several days in a row.

Since this book is all about implementable steps, let's create a plan and explanation here. With so many actionable ideas I don't want to overwhelm you with yet another tactic. The paragraph above is something that you can try at any point to experience hunger pains. Another option is to purposely postpone eating a full meal until dinner. Do not over indulge on this one meal, just eat like you learned in other areas of the book. The goal is to postpone eating until dinner for 3-4 days in a row after a month or two of implementing the other things. Because of the hungry feeling, I don't want you to start on this step and fail and then quit and not try anything else. Everyone is different and certain tips throughout the book will resonate better with you than others. My main goal for you by limiting your food for a few days, especially after a month of your body already adapting to the smaller meal portions, is to try and shrink your stomach. At some point in your life, two slices of pizza was enough for you to fill full. As time went on, you could now eat 6 slices and three sodas. The reason you can do that is because your stomach physically gets bigger. That means you have to fit more food in there to get that literal "I'm going to burst my stomach is so full from the unlimited buffet" feeling. We need to give our stomach time to shrink so that less food will give us the sensation of being full. There can be some uncomfortable hunger feelings if you do this method, so the following paragraph has some tips on how to alleviate them.

Here are a few ways out of some of the discomfort without actually eating a bunch of food all at once. You can eat 2 walnuts or 4-5 almonds when you feel hunger pains before your designated meal. The point of this delayed meal is to shrink the stomach and learn to embrace feeling a little hungry. Sometimes I am amazed that if I just eat a few nuts or half a banana or something equally small but high in calories, just how nicely it cuts my hunger cravings. Another strategy is to put ½ a teaspoon (not tablespoon) or a pinch of sugar into a glass of water. Wait, I can hear you say, you said sugar is the devil. Well, your brain is craving some sugar and if you just drink water or add artificial sweetener then in 10 minutes your brain says I'm hungry again. By adding that little bit of sugar and drinking that glass of water, the stomach will be stimulated and think it's been fed and the brain will get a taste of sugar and turn off the hunger signals for another hour or more. You tricked them both, good job. It's just water, so the body absorbs it quickly, but I would still recommend drinking only 8 ounces at a time so you don't overstretch the stomach.

21 BETTER TO EAT MORE AT BREAKFAST, LUNCH OR DINNER

I'm a proponent of having most of your calories for the day at breakfast and lunch. That way, you have the rest of the afternoon, including exercise and walking for some people, to use up the calories before bed. If we eat ½ our day's calories at the end of the day, we just tend to store it at night. You still need to eat something for dinner, but it could be light like fruit or a salad. Let me bring back that hunger pain again. If you had a big lunch, you may not get that hunger sensation again until 7 pm and if you just feed it a little, then you stopped the craving without having a gigantic meal. The evening, especially watching TV, is one of the easiest ways to mindlessly eat. I'm sure we all ate a whole bag of chips or popcorn or a gigantic bowl of ice cream while watching TV and then said afterward, "Uh oh I didn't mean to do that."

Night time is the best time to experience those hunger pains. Either deal with it until breakfast or feed it with a piece of fruit or something low in calories just so you can make it to bed. This is a nice way to cut calories, lose weight a little quicker and if you make it a lifestyle choice that only gets broken 20% of the time, you might just find it's a nice way to maintain a healthy weight too.

22 UNDERSTANDING ORGANIC FOOD LABELS

Most of us have bought something at the grocery store labeled as "organic." If you have, you'll want to pay attention here. It turns out labeling foods "organic" is trickier than you think. The word "organic" is becoming little more than a money-maker for corporations who want to jump on the "healthy" bandwagon. In fact, the FDA and USDA, which are the very agencies that are supposed to be protecting the organic food supply, are intensely active in its adulteration.

For example, did you know that a "certified organic" product can actually have a mix of organic and conventional ingredients? It's true. In fact, under the law, you could manufacture "organic beer" with completely conventional hops, label it "USDA Certified Organic" and charge a premium price for it -- hops are allowed to be non-organic under USDA Certified Organic products. This may have changed by the time you are reading this.

As Farm Wars puts it: "It's like putting gasoline in a glass of pure water and charging a premium for that water because it only contains 30 percent of the contaminant. 30 percent contamination is probably better than 100 percent, but would you want to drink it? The whole glass of water is poisoned due to the gasoline, yet the companies selling this product would like you to believe that because it contains pure water it is good."

How To Read Organic Labels:

If you're going to buy organic, it's important that you know what the different labels mean. There are several different organic labels out there, but only one relates directly to foods: the USDA Organic Seal. This seal is your best assurance of organic quality. Growers and manufacturers of organic products bearing the USDA seal have to meet the strictest standards of any of the currently available organic labels.

Products labeled "100% Organic" must contain only organically produced ingredients.

Products labeled "Certified Organic" must contain at least 95% organic ingredients.

Products labeled "Made with Organic Ingredients" can contain anywhere between 70 to 95% organic ingredients. So in order to get your money's worth when buying organic, make sure you are buying food with the label "100% USDA Organic."

23 WHEN IS THE BEST TIME TO EXERCISE?

Have you ever wondered what time of the day you should exercise? Believe it or not, working out at different times of the day accomplishes different results. Here is a list of benefits from exercising in the morning and exercising in the afternoon:

==================
MORNING BENEFITS:
==================

- More likely to stick to your exercise routine
- Better moods and less tension throughout the day
- Better mind-set for food intake
- Improvements in sleep patterns and cognitive function

====================
AFTERNOON BENEFITS:
====================

- Less chance of injury
- Increased respiratory capacity
- Less chance of sleep deprivation from rising early
- Greater improvement in sleep patterns and cognitive function

24 TESTOSTERONE AND HOW TO MAXIMIZE IT FOR EXERCISE

Testosterone is the hormone responsible for the sex drive, aggression (think those who take steroids or the feistiness of male teenagers) and can help build muscle bigger and faster. Testosterone cycles throughout the day normally in men and women but the rate differs for each person. For those who want to maximize the benefits from exercise or don't have a lot of time but want the best results in the time they do have, then this tip is for you. When deciding what time of day to exercise (morning, afternoon or evening), consciously think about when your sex drive peaks in the day. For some when they wake up they would be more ready to 'do it' than in the evening. If that it is you, then go work out in the morning and get that free testosterone boost. Attack the gym when your body's natural testosterone spikes to get that little extra boost in the workout.

Even though you can see that there are some specific benefits to working out at different times of the day, the most important thing is that you exercise regularly, no matter what time it is. Find a time when you can exercise for 30 to 60 minutes at least 3 to 4 times a week. Seriously, if you have never really tried aerobic exercise on any kind of regular schedule then don't feel bad if all you can muster is 10 minutes. Just stick with 10 minutes several times a week and add an extra 5 minutes every week. Read on for my cardio and weight lifting blueprints.

25 PERSONAL BLUEPRINT - CARDIO:

When I first started working out with cardio on a regular basis, I was 27 years old. That's not to say I didn't go to the gym or hike Colorado mountain trails, but I wasn't consistent. Running on a treadmill, and anywhere really, was tough on my shins. Maybe I needed to hire a coach to evaluate my running patterns to help with that, but I never did. What did I do? What changed my lazy patterns?

My family history of heart disease and diabetes finally got me serious about my own heart health. If I'm being vulnerable with you, a divorce was also a reason I got involved more consistently. Nothing like the emotional stress of divorce and the upheaval of life to get a bit stressed and what's better than a natural stress reliever like exercise. An added motivation was I needed to get my body in tiptop shape for attracting the ladies again. Seriously though, when going through an emotional turmoil like a divorce, it is very important to take care of your physical health as well as your mental wellbeing, especially if kids are involved. Personally I went to a counselor and studied some good books to work through the whole thing. Listen to my podcast, A Doctor's Perspective, and you can hear licensed marriage and family therapists, life-divorce coaches and PhD counselors discuss a wide array of topics. They recommended some great books and they can be found in each episode's show notes.

I started out on an elliptical machine. I love these machines because there is no stress on the knees, no bouncing, no jarring and it is just a smooth gliding motion that will hopefully translate into me not having bad knees when I'm old. The main drawback is that the cardio benefits will take a little extra effort, be it faster speed or longer time on it. A trick on the elliptical is to actually spend $2/3^{rd}$ of the time pedaling/gliding in the reverse direction (as if you were running backwards). It engages more hamstrings and is a little harder and better, in my opinion. When I started with a goal to do more heart healthy exercise, I was on the machine with a book, facing a TV at the gym with music in my ears. After about 6 minutes, I was still so bored and winded that I quit. Next day, I did the same thing, and the next day and the next. After a month I was up to 15 minutes without stopping. Reading and music continued to be my staples to get through the workout. Truthfully, I didn't push myself as hard while reading but my goal was to reach those set minutes. My thoughts were that I was not going to go from lounging on a Saturday to marathon finisher in 4 months, so I just took my time and built the habit and routine of exercise. Once I made it to 30 minutes and had a month or two under my belt, my body was adapted to it and, more importantly, my brain and motivation were adequate.

Knowing that I was not pushing hard enough with a book or cell phone in my hand, I purposely put my book down and increased my glide speed for one minute. Remember to adjust the difficulty of the machine when going fast otherwise it will feel quite awkward. I'm not saying to work so hard that it feels like climbing a mountain, but hard enough to feel some resistance when you pedal. After going close to my full speed for one minute, I would take a few minutes to recover and read and then do it again. This is actually called interval training and one of the best ways to get in shape quick. (I have a whole hack on interval training.)

One month I decided I wanted to do a 5k every time I got on the elliptical. It took a little longer than 40 minutes and I was bummed by that. I didn't want to be at the gym that long every day. (I was going to the gym 5-6 days a week at this point in my life- it was 2 minutes from the office on the way home.) So, I set the book down, put on 120 bpm (beats per minute) music, stared at the TV and pushed myself to lower my time until my 5k was less than 30 minutes. I think my best was 22 minutes. After reaching that milestone, I backed off and went back to my now normal 30 minutes on the machine each day. I am writing all this because I want you to be inspired and motivated. I did it and so can you.

26 PERSONAL BLUEPRINT - WEIGHTLIFTING

A word about weigh tlifting. Each time I went to the gym, I would do at least 6 different weigh tlifting exercises. I would vary the routine by using machines, dumbbells, and cable machines. Some days I would use a lot of weight and do my best to get 10 reps (repetitions) on each exercise. Some days I would do a weight that was only a little challenging but I would do 18 reps. Varying the weight encourages different muscle fibers to grow and puts different healthy strains on ligaments and tendons. I'm not training for big muscles, just stronger healthier muscles as well as joint stability. Truth be told, I do not even do two sets very often. I would do my 10 reps and immediately move on to the next exercise. No 30 second break, no talking and no looking at pretty girls (which most hate by the way), just one exercise after the other.

A quick rant: guys who cut normal shirts into that gaping armpit to waist sleeveless style look obnoxious to me. I also don't understand why guys can wear a full shirt and shorts to their knee and women roll up in the gym with a bra and spandex granny panties. Am I right? Rant over.

By not taking a break between weigh tlifting exercises, my heart rate stayed high and I felt like walking to the next machine or setting up the next barbell was break enough. A lot of people will scoff at not doing two sets, or not concentrating on two muscle groups and working them 10 different ways each day. Your criticism is noted and respectfully ignored. Exercise however you want, but this guide is set up for gym newbies and those who are intimidated and have no idea where to start but are ready to take that first step. Now there were days that I would do a more traditional workout, but I was going 6 days a week and I had other things to do besides spending all evening at the gym. In and out in 45 minutes or less is my goal. It's about being consistent and I've gained a lot of strength, confidence and look more attractive over the years because of it.

Most gyms have an area with a set amount of machines to train every muscle group. Maybe a goal for you is to do each machine (less than 12 machines usually) with at least 10 reps and 1 set. After every 4 machines, drink some water and then bang out the next 4. This might be a good way to develop a routine without being overwhelmed with all the options. If that is too many then just do half. Staff are more than willing to show you how to use any machine that you are unfamiliar with and might even recommend the top 6 that you could start with for maximum results.

Also, if you do a slow controlled motion at a safe weight, you should be able to minimize risk of injury while slowing still getting the gains. A safe weight for someone going from master couch potato to new gym membership is pretty easy to figure out. Put the pin on 10 pounds and do the exercise. Increase the weight until you feel resistance and it takes about 30% effort on your end to push it up. For example: If you were on a bicep curl machine loaded with 10 pounds and you could lift it up with zero effort then you should add 5 or 10 pounds. Now when you lift it you might feel your muscles actually engage and it takes some effort to bend your elbow. This could be that 30% effort and so is a good weight to start with. If you want to be extra diligent, bring a small note pad or use your phone to record the machine/exercise, the date, the weight you used, how many reps and sets you accomplished. Now you have proof of what you did and something to compare with a month from now. Did your weights stay the same or improve, and by how much? By the end of the month, if you haven't had to increase the amount of weight yet, go ahead and go one plate heavier and see how that feels. My guess is you are able to do it, but you just didn't want to yet.

27 WEIGHT LIFT BOOSTER AND SCHEDULE:

To maximize your efforts, do the following. When doing a chest exercise for example, we typically push the bar out at a nice smooth rate and then quickly bring it back to our chest. My goal for you is to try one of two ways presented to change up your routine and see faster results. 1.) Push the weight out at your normal speed, but when you are bringing the machine back to the starting position, I want you to go slow and take 4 seconds. We call this 'working the negative'. It's almost guaranteed to give you more strength in a shorter amount of time than the usual way. 2.) When you push the weight out and return the weight to the starting position, go slow and take 4 seconds each way. Good luck reaching 10 reps because it makes you tired in a hurry. I like mixing both of these styles into my weekly routine. At first, you don't have to do this method for your entire session, just try it on two exercises. Eventually you could work your way into doing method 1 for an entire session and, two sessions later, do method 2 for the entire time.

Basic Weekly Weight Lifting Schedule Blueprint

Day 1: 2 sets of 10 with normal weight,
Day 2: 1 set of 10 high resistance with Method 2,
Day 3: 1 set of 18 with normal weight,

Day 4: 2 sets of 10 with normal weight with Method 1,
Day 5: Mix it up however you want. Do your favorite exercises with your favorite methods. Also, learn one new exercise.

Blueprint Wrap-up:

Before you know it, you have reached a 30 minute cardio goal and you built a nice muscle routine. Did you know that muscle burns more calories than fat all day long? Did you know that females will not look like male body builders if they lift weights and the super muscular women on magazines focus on gaining muscle by eating a certain way and staying in the gym 2-4 hours per day? Ladies, put away those myths and fears about looking like a dude, it won't happen. Just do some weights, get stronger, build some muscle and burn more fat all day long. Trust me, the average man and woman won't even look like one of those athletes on workout/cardio videos even if they do the video series for the 90 days they recommend. Living in China has showed me it's possible to be a healthy weight at all ages but with our sedentary, carb-filled western lifestyles, it makes our journey more difficult. Do your best to stick to your schedule. You can do it. Take action - get healthier!

28 PERSONALIZED CALORIE CONSUMPTION CALCULATOR

Are you confused about the percentages of fat vs. protein vs. carbs you should have in your diet? Do you find yourself asking, "How many calories should I eat?" or "Can I eat more every day if I exercise?", the ever popular "How long will it take to lose 10 pounds?" and "Are there any ways to bio-hack and speed up my health goals?"

Have no fear, all these questions will be answered in this chapter.

A BMI chart shows your height, weight, and a sliding scale of your body fat that ranges from underweight, normal, overweight, and obese based on all these numbers. (https://www.nhlbi.nih.gov/health/educational/lose_wt/BMI/bmi_tbl.htm) Obviously, a 5 foot person who weighs 180 pounds is not going to be as healthy as a 6 foot 5" person with the same weight. The easiest way I can help you is for you to follow along and do some math with me. You can do it. You just need to follow my example step by step and plug in your height and weight.

Step 1

Below are three formulas. Each one will give you a different amount of total calories that your body would burn if you did normal activities like walk around your house, drive a car, digest food, and just survive. As you are probably aware, just staying alive by digesting food, rebuilding cells, and thinking requires your body to burn calories all day long.

One of the formulas calculates a Lean Body Mass number. I will show you three ways to find that number so you can use an average for the main formula. I highly suggest doing each of the formulas for yourself and then taking the average of them as your goal for calorie consumption. This will allow you to understand higher or lower calorie consumption for you so you can still be within your personalized limits.

Step 2

Finding the base amount of calories that your body will burn per day is a good start for most people. If you eat only that many calories per day versus what you eat now, the weight would melt off you.

I expect you to exercise. It boosts your mood, has antidepressant attributes, gives you energy throughout the day, helps you handle stress and anxiety better, can help you think better, have more mental clarity, and improves your sleep and sex life. You can read my own personal exercise journey and my tips in Chapters 25 and 26.

Let me bust a weight loss myth about exercise: I can eat more or reward myself because I worked out. It takes nearly an hour of walking to burn off a 12oz soda. Stop rewarding yourself with a big dessert for working hard all week at the gym because you just negated it. I want you to be aware that it takes a shockingly long time to burn 200 calories and we sometimes sabotage ourselves without even being conscious of it.

Sure, you need more protein calories (and a little more carbs) if you are trying to bulk up for a weightlifting competition, but I'm talking about someone looking to lose weight by starting to exercise and then rewards that good behavior by eating chips and salsa because they 'earned it'. Is there anything inherently wrong with eating chips and salsa? No, but if you eat a full bag, that's a step back on your journey.

The battle with the scale is won at the dinner table while exercise is for cardiovascular health and other health benefits, not so much for weight loss. With that being said, I do have some seemingly contradictory information for you. One side effect of exercise is that you are able to eat a little bit more and still be in a healthy range for you. Step 2's formulas will show you just how much.

The formula to find out how many calories you can eat to just survive and maintain your weight goal is called the "Activity Multiplier" And this is important for long-term weight maintenance. At first you may want to stick to the average calorie consumption found from the three formulas so you can maximize weight loss. At some point in the future, you will be at your ideal weight and will be continue to exercise out of habit and joy. You should stop losing weight and this Activity Multiplier will give you a new calorie consumption goal so you maintain your weight, not lose more.

Step 3

This last step is optional and has two formulas. For those who have been overeating for a long time, a sudden drop in calories will be too hard to handle and they will quit. I want you to succeed in your health goals so I have a strategy to help you out.

The second formula in step 3 will give you guidance on how to determine how much protein vs. carbs vs. fat you should eat. I briefly cover intermittent fasting and how this could be a bio-hack to jump start improvements in your blood work and make your clothes feel baggier than ever.

Formula One: The first formla is a way to slowly reduce the calories you currently eat so you don't feel like you're starving. This helps with the mental aspect of losing weight and being hungry. Your stomach has been stretched out from over eating and needs time to shrink back to a more normal size. Remember at some point in life two slices of pizza, a beer, and a brownie made you feel stuffed, but now it's four slices, two beers, one soda and three brownies... all that food had to fit in your stomach somehow.

Formula Two: Some people follow diets that talk about a percentage of your food being a certain type of macronutrient and others talk about grams of food. For instance, a ketogenic diet (or just a lower carb diet in general) is a diet with X% of Fat, Y% of Protein and Z% of Carbs. If you look at nutrition labels, you will see some percentages are based on a 2000 calorie diet. That's great, but you problaby aren't on a 2000 calorie diet.

These formulas will help you have a complete customized plan just for you. You will be able to calculate how many calories you are consuming from each macronutrient. As a bonus, you will learn an easier way to calculate everything from a nutrional label by tallying up the grams of everything you eat. If your diet plan says you should only eat 20% carbs, you can calculate how many calories you should eat per day, figure out what 20% of the total is, and how many grams of carbs it would take to max that out. Now all you have to do is consult the label for grams. It doesn't get much easier than adding grams all day.

Time to Break Out your Calculators and Find Your Calorie Goals

STEP 1: The three formulas for optimal calorie consumption

1. Mifflin-St. Jeor equation

    10x(kg) + (6.25*cm) - (5*your age) + 5 (for men)=
    10x(kg) + (6.25*cm) - (5*your age) - 161 (for women)=

2. Harris Benedict equation

    66 + (6.23* weight pounds) + (12.7*height in total inches) - (6.8*your age) male
    65 + (4.35* weight pounds) + (14.7*height in total inches) - (4.7*your age) female

3. Katch McArdle equation along with the 3 Lean Body Mass Formulas (below)

    370 + (21.6*lean body mass eLPM)

The "3 Lean Body Mass" Formula (eLPM) for the Katch McArdle Formula are:

A) The Boer Formula:

   Men: eLBM = 0.407 weight (kg) + 0.267 height (cm) - 19.2
   Women: eLBM = 0.252 weight (kg) + 0.473 height (cm) - 48.3

   Boer P. "Estimated lean body mass as an index for normalization of body fluid volumes in man." *Am J Physiol* 1984; 247: F632-5

B) The James Formula:

   Men: eLBM = 1.1 weight (kg) – 128 (weight (kg) / height

$(cm))^2$
Women: eLBM = 1.07 weight (kg) − 148 (weight $(kg)/height (cm))^2$

Absalom AR, Mani V, DeSmet T, et al. "Pharmacokinetic models for propofol-defining and illuminating the devil in the detail." *Br J Anaesth* 2009; 103:26-37

C) The Hume Formula:

Men: eLBM = 0.32810 weight (kg) + 0.33929 height (cm) - 29.5336
Women: eLBM = 0.29569 weight (kg) + 0.41813 height (cm) - 43.2933

Hume, R "Prediction of lean body mass from height and weight." *J Clin Pathol.* 1966 Jul; 19(4):389-91

http://www.calculator.net/lean-body-mass-calculator.html?ctype=metric&cage=25&csex=m&cheightfeet=5&cheightinch=10&cpound=160&cheightmeter=175&ckg=70.5&x=68&y=9

I will illustrate each formula for a 34-year old guy who is 5 foot 7 inches and 155 pounds.

First things first, You need to convert your weight from pounds (lb) to kilograms (kg) and your height from feet and inches to centimeters (cm).

The * symbol means multiply.
The / symbol means divide.

Pounds to kilogram (kg): *XX Pounds * 0.4536= weight in kg*

Example: 155 lb * 0.4536 = 70.31 kg

Feet and inches to centimeters (cm):

First convert your feet to inches: _X_ Feet * 12= _Y_ inches.
Now add Y inches to the remainder of your height

(in our example, the guy is 5 ft 7 inches so it would be Y+7=Z). Let's call that total _Z.
_Z_ * 2.54= height in cm.

*Example: 5 ft 7 inch male. 5ft * 12 = 60 inches. 60 inches + 7 inches = 67 inches*
*67 inches * 2.54= 170.18 CM*

<u>WRITE DOWN the KG and the CM because you will be using these a lot in the rest of the formulas.</u>

Let's find out your **Lean Body Mass Numbers***, create an average, and then do the three Optimal Calorie Consumption formulas. Remember, just follow along and put your height and weight in the example instead of mine. You don't have to remember algebra because I will walk you through it step by step. People say if you give something away for free, they won't really value it and probably won't follow through with whatever advice was given. However, if you pay something for that advice, even if it's a small amount or it's paid by spending time and effort, the person will value it and act on the advice given. So please, take out a pencil and paper and figure out your numbers.*

(If you are female, use the female formulas.)

A) **The Boer Formula:** {If female use = 0.252 weight (kg) + 0.473 height (cm) - 48.3 }

Men: eLBM = 0.407 * weight (kg) + 0.267 * height (cm) - 19.2

0.407 * 70.31 = *28.62*
0.267* 170.18 = *45.44*
28.62 + 45.44 - 19.2 = **54.86**

B) **The James Formula:** {If female use= 1.07 weight (kg) – 148 (weight (kg) / height (cm))^2 }

Men: eLBM = 1.1 * weight (kg) − 128 * (weight (kg) / height (cm))2

> 1.1 * 70.31 = *77.34*
> Kg/cm 70.31 / 170.18 = 0.413 (type it in your calculator just as you see it here)
> The ^{2} means you multiple 0.413 by itself. 0.413 * 0.413 = *0.17*
> 128 * 0.17 = *21.76*
> 77.34 - 21.76 = **55.58**

C) **The Hume Formula**: {If female use= 0.29569 weight (kg) + 0.41813 height (cm) - 43.2933}

Men: eLBM = 0.32810 * weight (kg) + 0.33929 * height (cm) - 29.5336

> 0.32810 * 70.31 = *23.07*
> .33929 * 170.18 = *57.74*
> 23.07 + 57.74 − 29.5336 = **51.28**

AVERAGE of the LEAN BODY MASS FORMULA
 Add the three totals together. 54.86 + 55.58 + 51.28 = 161.69
 Now divide by three and you get the average. 161.69 / 3 = **53.90**

You did a great job doing all that math to find that one number.
Let's continue to the moment we've all been waiting for...

Calculating the Three Formulas for Optimal Calorie Consumption

1) **Mifflin-St. Jeor equation**

   10*(kg) + (6.25*cm) - (5*your age) + 5 (for men) =

10*(kg) + (6.25*cm) - (5*your age) - 161 (for women) =

Our Example: Men (10 * 70.31) + (6.25 * 170.18) - (5 * 34) + 5=
10 * 70.31 = 703.1   6.25 * 170.18 = 1063.625   5 * 34 = 70
703.1 + 1063.625 - 70 + 5 = **1602**

2) Harris Benedict equation

Male: 66 + (6.23 * weight pounds) + (12.7 * height in total inches) - (6.8* age)
Female: 65 + (4.35 * weight pounds) + (14.7 * height in total inches) - (4.7* age)

Our example: Men
66 + (6.23*155) + (12.7*76) – (6.8*34) =
6.23 * 155 = 965.65   12.7 * 76 = 965.2   6.8 * 34 = 231.2
66 + 965.65 + 965.2 - 231.2 = **1766**

3) Katch McArdle equation

370 + (21.6 * lean body mass)

370 + (21.6 * 53.9) =
21.6 * 53.9 = 1164
370 + 1164 = **1534**

AVERAGE of all Three Formulas for Optimal Calorie Consumption

For a 34 year old, 5 ft 7 in and 155 pound male
1602 Miffin-St Jeor + 1766 Harris Benedict + 1534 Katch McArde = 4902
4902 / 3 = 1634

1634 Calories burned on average each day

Step 2: Activity Multiplier

We should all be exercising at least 3-4 times per week. Lifting weights, running, walking with speed, elliptical machine, and sports are all exercise. This activity multiplier allows you to increase your daily calorie limit and assumes only hours spent doing exercise—not an hour at the gym if you really only ran for 35 minutes and talked the rest of the time. It also requires you to be honest with yourself on the intensity of your workout. A 55-year-old woman will have different measurements that classify a workout as moderate compared to an 18-year-old male. The 18 year old will need a higher heart rate to be in the moderate intensity level than the 55 year old female. To account for age and sex related differences, you have to be very honest with yourself when choosing your Activity Multiplier.

Do you only work out for a total of 2 hours a week but you run 7 miles in 30 minutes and can hardly breathe? Well, maybe you should do moderate exercise. Do you walk 6 hours a week but at a slow pace and you are only 35 years old? Then maybe you should do light exercise. Do you understand what I am illustrating? Don't go just by the time spent; factor in how intense you are working out as well. The secret sauce for success is to go moderate or intense for however many hours per week you exercise. If you are already spending your time exercising, why not maximize the effort.

This book gives you blueprints on how to go from a couch potato to being able to exercise for 30 minutes without stopping. I realize you can't go from 5 hours a day of TV watching to doing a stair climber machine for 20 minutes in day one. It's a slow process to ramp up, but it can be done. Be easy on yourself, and be honest when figuring out which Activity Multiplier you pick.

Remember, the multiplier allows you to consume more calories per day. If you eat more calories and quit exercising, don't be surprised when weight loss stops. At some point you will be at your target weight goals and you may want to stick to this higher calorie amount so you don't keep shrinking.

Activity Multiplier Chart

Multiplier	Exercise Intensity
1.2	desk job, little exercise
1.375	1-3 hours per week light exercise
1.55	3-5 hours per week moderate exercise
1.75	5-6 hours a week intense exercise
1.9	two hours every day strenuous

Your new calorie intake based on activity level is found by multiplying the Activity Multiplier you choose on the left in the above chart by the average of the three optimal calorie consumption formulas you calculated earlier.

For our example: this male walks at a moderate pace 4 times a week for 4 hours total (let's call that light exercise) and he does 90 minutes of moderate elliptical activity (moderate exercise). I am a little more conservative on my estimates and would rather eat fewer calories instead of more just in case I don't stick to my normal routine for a month. Based on time alone, the moderate exercise would seem to be an appropriate multiplier (1.55), but 70% of the time involves light exercise. Therefore, I would use the 1.375 multiplier.

Activity Multiplier: 1634 calories * 1.375 = 2246

Step 3: Slow Drop in Calories and Macronutrient Ratios

Slow Drop in Calories

Step A: This step requires you to know how many calories you are actually eating right now on average. How can you figure this number out? Easy! Almost everything we eat has a nutritional label on it that states the calories per serving. If you eat out a lot, check the restaurants' websites for calorie information on their dishes. Don't forget to record all drinks: milk, juice, soda, alcohol, etc. You just need to record the total calories for about five days. The internet has a ton of information on how many calories are in a cup of asparagus, rib eye steak, and sweet peas, etc. I think the most time consuming but also eye opening experience is to actually measure out just how many peas/ carrots/ potato's fit into a cup. Do that for five days and you can see how it will impact your eating habits for the rest of your life. Sometimes the hardest part of tracking food is honestly not knowing how much you ate. Think about a bowl of cereal. I typically just fill it ¾ full. One day, I measured it and I was amazed; I could have just eaten a candy bar or two donuts and had the same amount of sugar.

As this is a time consuming way of measuring, I would like to suggest a different method.

There is a great app called MyFitnessPal® (and a website) that has the nutritional information on everything from your favorite burrito at a fast food chain, to a cup of rice, frozen pizza, cappuccino (and the flavored cream you put in it), broccoli, candy bars, smoothie, two whiskey shots, six ounces of chicken breast (baked, fried, steamed), all the dishes at major chain restaurants, and on and on. I prefer this method because once you go through the hassle of finding it once, it will be saved for future use. You can record things accurately like breakfast, lunch, snacks and dinner. You can even record the exercise you do. You can pair it with a workout app or even in the app itself, and it will even let you set weight loss goals and a time frame. Then it gives you graphs and more information to tell you that you ate 2,500 calories but you ran and burned 300 calories so you can eat XYZ calories more than usual and still meet your goal of 10 pounds lost in 8 weeks. It will also break down how many carbs, protein, and fat in your food for the day. This will be important and convenient for monitoring, as discussed in the second half of Step 3.

Whether you use paper or an app, you have to know how much food you consume. What exactly is a cup of broccoli? Is it three little branches stuffed in a cup the right measurement or should we treat broccoli as if it was the texture of mashed potatoes? Corn and peas fit nicely in a cup, but a chicken breast doesn't. When cooking, you need to be able to accurately measure how much of each item you eat. Otherwise, you are guessing and you may guess high or low; either way, this is not an accurate way to track. A better way is to weigh your food on a food scale. You should use one that can show grams and ounces. Depending on the app you use, the developer may have chosen one or the other. Honestly, grams are easier because there is no guessing like there is with ounces, but it's your choice. Now you can look at what an official serving of broccoli is and measure out the exact amount.

Alright, you have just tracked five normal days of eating and drinking. What is your total amount of calories per day? Are you surprised that you could eat 4,200 calories or that the meal you had at lunch was 1,600 calories though it seemed like a small portion? Where dishes are hiding calories (and salt)? Is it any wonder you can't lose weight? Write down the total calories per day and then divide it by the amount of days you tracked it for. That is your average daily calorie consumption.

Example: 3,500 + 2,800 + 3,900 + 2,700 + 4,200 = 17,10017,100 / 5 = **3,420 average per day**

Step B: We need to reduce your calorie intake so you can lose weight. If we just immediately went from eating over 3,400 calories per day to the recommended values you calculated a few pages ago, you would quit. You will be so hungry all day and will have to deal with the psychological warfare of wanting to eat and being hungry but knowing you shouldn't. It's quite a mess and it sets you up for failure as well as guilt for not meeting your goals, and possibly depression if you are prone to it. Let's avoid all these negative outcomes and try a different method other than, "On Monday, I am only eating 1,700 calories (instead of 3,400) and I won't stop until I lose 25 pounds."

Gradual Reduction of Calories Method

We already know that the guy in our example has a goal of eating between 1,634 to 2,246 calories per day. We also know he is eating and drinking 3,420 calories on average per day. 3,420 minus 2,246 is 1,174 calories that he needs to stop consuming every day for a long time. Let imagine he has 25 pounds to lose for this section so he has to get his calorie intake under control.

Week 1

For the *first week,* he only needs to consume 250 fewer calories than normal. He can log all the food he eats /drinks on the website or app or paper and when he reaches 3,170, he must stop eating and drinking for the day. Remember that 250 calories could easily be drinking one less soda per day or a small version of that sugar coffee drink or one less beer or one less candy bar. Maybe you just need to sip that soda for an extra hour or two so you can trick yourself into never missing it. I think you get the idea. For this entire week, you make a small change that will allow you to adapt to fewer calories.

Week 2

Week two, you will reduce by another 250 calories: from 3,170 to 2,920 calories is your new daily calorie consumption. Again, you will need to find ways to reduce your total intake. This time you might cut out juice and milk in the morning or only order a small portion of French fries. Remember, you have weeks of data on that app. Go through it and you should start seeing trends about the time of day you tend to eat snacks. Maybe you can go for a walk or drink water instead of eating during that trouble zone. Perhaps you are noticing that you eat fast food more often on certain days and could plan ahead the night before and bring leftovers to work.

If you feel like you are doing great and are not struggling with reducing your food and drinks, then maybe you can reduce your calorie intake by 250 every 4-5 days. However, if you aren't comfortable with that, just reduce it by 250 every week until you reach your Optimal Activity Based Calorie Consumption Total. In our example, it will take five weeks for our guy to only consume 2,246 per day. He is patient and ok with this because he is experiencing a long-term lifestyle change and not a fad diet to lose weight as fast as possible. He might even notice the scale dip since he started exercising while reducing his daily calories by 250 per day. How exciting is that? All the while he is letting his stomach shrink and creating healthy habits. He has daily small victories that build up his dieting self-esteem and has been making positive changes in his food choices.

BONUS: I have one more trick for you to maximize your calorie to weight loss ratio. We already established a tactic to get you to your activity-based daily calorie consumption amount. If you want to reduce your weight faster, by all means you can just eat the normal calorie amount without the activity multiplier. However, you will probably be hungry and cheat. I could cheat with a brownie or a few spoonfuls too many of peanut butter to make some celery more palatable. My hack is to target somewhere in the middle of the minimum and maximum of your appropriate range.

Here's how to do it. Take the total activity level calorie consumption calories and cut 15%. The difference lets you have 15% more calorie restriction to lose weight and be fuller than just sticking to the minimum calorie requirements.

$$2246 * .15 = 337 \quad 2246 - 337 = 1909$$

This logic is a little off, but it illustrates the point well enough. Eating too few calories is tough and I want you to reach your goals. Therefore, I encourage using the activity multiplier so you can eat more food. However, it's nice to see results quicker so doing this 15% trick is my little secret bonus. We know a pound of fat is about 3,500 calories. Assuming you reduce your activity-based calories by 15% (in our example, 337 calories) then you could lose an extra pound every 10.4 days. 3500 / 337 = 10.4

Macronutrient Ratios

The market is flooded with diet, weight loss, and exercise books. You can find Paleo, vegetarian, vegan, keto, Atkins, modified keto, vegetarian with seafood, low carb, high protein, gluten free, soup only, count your calories as points, juice everything, intermittent fasting, and the list could go on. Every diet has good intentions and usually some unexpected consequences. I'm not saying the consequences are fatal, only that you may find that if you are on a soup only diet (yes, you lose 15 pounds in a month), you gain it all back when you eat real food again. Some diets demonize certain foods or food groups and expect you to never eat the culprit again. Guess what? That rarely works and you end up craving it more, and when you finally break down, you never go back. Have you experienced that before?

I don't know what you have tried in the past or what you are currently trying. I will show you how to figure out how many grams of macronutrients equals calories. If you follow my suggestions or some other method that promotes an "eat XYZ amount of protein per day", you will know how to figure that out. You should have already calculated your Optimal Activity Based Caloric Consumption per day and now you can do some math and figure out how many grams and at what percent of your personal calorie amount you should eat to faithfully prescribe to a diet plan (and hopefully a lifestyle change) so you can reach your target goals.

What is a Macronutrient?

Feel free to Wikipedia® it for a deep dive into what they are. You can also read many books on all the subtleties of good oils, bad oils, healthiest protein, high glycemic index fruits, and so on. I will only give you a brief overview. There are three Macronutrients: Carbohydrates, Fat and Protein.

Protein

Protein can be lean or fat, dark or white, and some are healthier for you than others. Research always goes back and forth on whether you should eat egg yolks, but I don't' see an issue with it. If you are worried, maybe just eat ½ whites and ½ yolks. Deer and buffalo are some of the best meats around whereas beef and chicken thighs tend to get a bad reputation in the heart health community. You can eat protein from plants and vegetables as well, like quinoa. We even have protein powders and snack bars made of whey, chickpeas, vegan based, and more options if you have allergies. We have a wide array of options when it comes to protein. If you find that you need 100 grams of protein a day, don't sweat it; you don't have to consume it all as hamburgers and turkey breast. Protein shakes make a nice snack to keep you away from chips and candy while giving you a boost in energy and meeting your daily food requirements.

Protein can be thought of as fuel to maintain your muscles; if you want to grow muscles, you eat more protein. Many diets don't stress the need to eat enough protein and the body will actually break down protein easier than fat. That means you lose muscle mass for that first month on a diet instead of losing fat. The body does what's easiest to process. When you look at our ancestors, fat kept them alive in the long winters, not big muscles. I can't stress enough that you should eat adequate amounts of protein. (If you decide to do a ketogenic or modified Atkins type diet where the carbs are below 10% and the protein is around 20%, make sure you don't eat 30-40% protein because the body has a way of breaking down excess protein and then treats it like a carb. Those hidden protein carbs will sabotage you into ketosis.)

Carbohydrates

Carbohydrates can be anything from refined sugar, bread, pasta, potatoes, and all fruits. Some fruits contain way more sugar than others and if you eat too many, the body treats it like a candy bar. Sure, you get more nutrients, but the insulin response to the body is the same. There's a reason diabetics shouldn't eat an entire container of strawberries all at once.

Check online for charts about the carb content of different fruits and vegetables. The fancy term for this is a glycemic index and you will find that you can eat plenty of fruits and vegetables that are on the low side. A fruit like an avocado is quite good for you; it has low carbs and has an amazing amount of healthy oils.

We should all strive to eat a wide variety of fruits, vegetables, legumes, and grains. I think a diet with fewer carbs is an ideal way to live. This doesn't mean you can't have indulgences but we need to limit them and not eat them every day. Do yourself a favor and print off a list of low glycemic foods and bring it with you next time you shop.

Some people have a real gluten intolerance that gives them headaches and diarrhea if they eat it. Other people may find that they have some "weird" health symptoms, joint pains that barely subside, or always have low energy and fell sluggish; they actually feel so much better after a few weeks if they avoid gluten.

I prescribe to the idea of limiting the carbohydrates in our diet. We eat way too many desserts, rice, pasta, potatoes, and high sugar fruits. I believe this is why half the country is overweight and obese, and it explains the rise in overweight children in developing countries that are adopting a western fast food, processed food diet. You can find some great books and research linking high carb eating (60-70% or more of the diet) to diabetes, chronic joint pain, a lack of energy, arthritis, thyroid issues, and everyone's favorite obsession, high cholesterol and the clogging of arteries. There is growing evidence that when the science community was debating if high sugar or high fat were the culprit for heart disease, the fat people won, though they shouldn't have. Ever wonder why margarine is no longer touted as a great alternative to butter? Ever wonder why heart disease is continuing to rise even though millions take statins every day? Maybe, just maybe, when they started making everything low fat and adding sugar so you would eat the food, the high sugar consumption over the past few decades is the real reason for the heart health epidemic.

Sugar molecules have lots of sharp corners. When sugar floats in your arteries, it nicks the inner lining. The fat that is also circulating in the arteries is sticky and fills in those nicks. Remember the last time you got a scratch or cut on your arm and the skin around the cut became swollen and red? That is called inflammation and that actually occurs in the arteries as well. This process continues to worsen because we always have way to much sugar in our blood, nicks abound, fat accumulates, until one day you get a blocked artery. When people stick to a lower carb diet for a few months, their blood work tends to improve. If eating more healthy fat and limiting sugar/carbs was as evil as they would have you believe, the blood work should get worse... but it doesn't for many people.

I highly recommend getting a full blood workup before changing your diet, especially if it's based on macronutrient percentages. After three months of the new diet, get retested. Your doctor can compare what this new eating profile is doing for you. Some people find that eating more fat and restricted carbs is actually bad for their body and they need to stop. Others know that they have been cheating or not actually monitoring the type of food they eat (as in, they eat deep fried chicken everyday instead of grilled chicken breasts cooked in a little extra virgin olive oil). You can only deal with the data you have. Redo your blood work 3-4 times a year and make sure you are healthy on the inside not just artificially on the outside.

Carbohydrates are broken down and the body and brain like to use them in preference to anything else. It's very easy for the body to use and our processed food supplies it in high amounts.

Fat

We all know fat can be saturated and unsaturated, but what about hydrogenated, trans fat, polyunsaturated, and healthy oils? Coconut oils, MCT oils, extra virgin olive oils, nuts, omega fish oils (omega 3's and 6's), and a few more are healthy fats are the best to cook with, drizzle on salads and consume on a regular basis. Soybean, peanut, sunflower, vegetable oil, and many more are not considered desirable in the diet so you should limit them. You can also get naturally occurring fats from certain fruits, vegetables, and in fat/nutrient dense nuts.

Fat is typically the last thing the body wants to process for energy but it yields the most calories/energy per gram. If you have a habit of eating a jar of almonds and macadamia nuts, you will probably gain weight because one jar is about 1,000 extra calories. Nuts have their own delicious oils, which make them easy to overeat, but they are very calorie dense. One small handful of nuts a day is enough.

Also, I mentioned earlier about how restaurants hide calories, mainly by cooking in junk oil. One tablespoon is over 100 calories. The goal of the restaurant is to cook tasty food and not healthy food. Oil (and salt) will make just about any meal taste better. Fried chicken and fried fish are bad for you because the batter and the meat actually absorb oil, which will make you fat and increase your cholesterol. Just go on MyFitnessPal® and plug in baked chicken leg versus a fried leg and be ready to have your mind blown. Eating healthy fat is an entirely different scenario.

Tools to Help

The following are several strategies to experiment with on what percentage of each macronutrient profile you will follow. If you would rather not deal with any more math, the website http://www.keto-calculator.ankerl.com is amazing. They programmed the math for you so all you have to do is fill in what they tell you to. Near the bottom of the page, they break down the percentage of each macronutrient, what amount of calories you will eat of each, and how many grams. Plus, it has the activity multiplier, daily calorie intake, and gives you a range of protein you should eat based on your goals. You can also track what percentage of calories you would like to cut and it estimates how much weight you will lose each month. It's free too.

Calculations

| 1 gram of carb = 4 calories | 1 gram of protein = 4 calories | 1 gram of fat = 9 calories |

When calculating carbs, use this formula: Total Carbs − Fiber = Net Carbs

When determining a carb on a nutritional label, make sure to subtract the fiber amount from the total carb number. The result is Net Carbs, which is the number of grams we want to track in the carb macronutrient percentage.

Total Carbs – Fiber = Net Carbs
Total Carb 25 – Fiber 15 = 10 net carbs

If you want a normal range of **protein** to eat then you want about 0.8 grams of protein per kilogram of your weight. If you are more active, eat 1.0 grams of protein per kilogram of your weight. If you are extra active or building bigger muscles then you can eat 1.2 grams of protein per kilogram of your weight.

Example: Our guy (70.3 kg) has an active lifestyle and lifts weights

70.3 * 1.0 = 70 grams of protein to eat per day

Grams of protein to eat per kilogram you weigh each day
Normal range	0.8
Active lifestyle	1.0
Very Active or Building Muscles	1.2

Let's examine a good macronutrient profile.

Protein

First calculate how many grams of protein you need to eat per day with the above formula and then multiply that by 4 (calories). Then =divide that number by the total amount of calories you eat per day to get the percent of protein specific for you. (If you are reducing calories by 250 per week then redo these percentages and macronutrient breakdowns each week so you have the accurate amount.)

X grams of protein * 4 = Y calories from protein
Then Y / total calories (with activity) = __ percent of calories from protein

Example: Our guy needs 70 grams of protein.

70 * 4 = 280 calories   280 calories / 2246 = .1246
.1246 * 100 = **12.46%**

Our guy would eat 12.5% of his diet as protein = 70 grams = 280 Calories

Carbohydrates

Ketosis: If you are trying to be ketogenic, you should eat between 30-50 grams of carbs per day. That is actually quite difficult to do and tends to be only 5-10% of your daily calories. Again, a quick search online will give you information on recipes, calculators, support groups, how to, and everything else imaginable. I like the idea of keto and taking exogenous ketones and MCT oil, but I haven't experimented and studied =enough to talk much about it. The benefits I have read and experts discussing it on podcasts fascinates me and is worth learning more about. There are so many online resources that beginners can read and see for themselves. Do a quick calculation with an apple and an orange a day and you will quickly hit the carb limit. Though there are variations to the diet for carb intake, it's still hard. Eating this way has been to reduce insulin resistance, reduce seizures, has varying positive effects on cancer, supplies more efficient energy to the brain, and benefits Alzheimer's, epilepsy, depression, and migraines. Most of these studies are not definitive and some where only in rat models, which though promising, requires more research.

Ketosis macronutrient breakdown: Proteins 15-30% carbs 5-10% (30-50 grams) fat 60-75%

100 gram Method: There are online communities and websites dedicated to keeping your carbs around 100 grams or fewer per day for optimal results. It allows you to make wise fruit decisions whereas a keto or modified keto diet requires you to eliminate fruit to keep carb intake between 30-50 grams per day. This 100 grams of Carbs Method lets you have more choices in food but still requires you to be picky about how you satisfy that amount. Another benefit is that it will keep the low carb mood dip and mental fog from happening. Bottom line, lowering your carbs can help reverse diabetes, lower cholesterol, and triglycerides, so I suggest you try this method. Go online and print off a low glycemic index food list (fruit, veggies, grains, beans, legumes) and bring it with you when you shop, prepare food, and eat outside the home. After a few weeks, you will not have to check your food labels as much because the food will become familiar.

Carbohydrates: keep them low. 15-20% of your total calories or under 100 grams

$2{,}246 * .20 = 449$ calories $449 / 4 = 112$ grams
$2{,}246 * .175 = 393$ calories $393 / 4 = 98$ grams
$2{,}246 * .15 = 337$ calories $337 / 4 = 84$ grams

Fats are the remaining calories.

Protein 280 (12.5%) + Carbs 393 (17.5%) − 2,246 = 1,573 calories from Fat

1,573 / 9 = 175 grams of Fat

> Fat: the remainder of the calories.
> In our example: Fat is 70% of total calories:
> 1,573 calories, 175 grams

Personally I like the following macronutrient breakdown, which is a mix of the methods described. We allow more protein than the "grams of protein to eat" chart earlier, we keep the carbs low but with a little wiggle room, and we have more fat than a typical western diet. This way we can still allow our body to use the ketone to supply the bulk of our energy needs and reduce chronic inflammation. This also helps boost weight loss, but I also like it because it will help stop metabolic syndromes (diabetes, high blood pressure, high cholesterol).

Protein 23%   Carbohydrate 15%   Fat 62%

Let's quickly look at the total grams and calories represented with this final macronutrient breakdown.

Protein 23%	0.23 * 2,246 = 516 cal	516/4 = 129g
Carbs 15%	0.15 * 2,246 = 337 cal	337/9 = 37g
Fat 62%	0.62 * 2,246 = 1,392 cal	1,392/4 = 348g

BONUS

Intermittent Fasting Guide

Have you heard of intermittent fasting? It is all the rage right now in the bio-hacking realm. I'll give you a little theory about it and present a couple options of how to do it; it might enhance all the hard work you are about to embark upon. Fasting is not the same as dieting. With a fast, you are purposely not eating during certain parts of the day and only eating during a specific window of time, but you are still eating the same amount of calories. Some people find it difficult to eat all the calories in the predetermined window of time, but they are in the minority. I think the biggest hurdle is the idea of purposely skipping breakfast or dinner every day and the 'hunger' that may ensue. There are others who fear being hungry and I would say drink more water, tea, or coffee when you feel hungry and you'll be alright. Seriously though, if you get the shakes or lightheaded or extra irritable, then you are a bad candidate for fasting, so quit. For the rest of us brave enough to embrace a little tummy grumbling, let's read a few quick facts about it and lay out two plans.

This isn't a research paper so don't expect to find references for some of these claims. A quick search on intermittent fasting will show you similar information with references that go into a lot more detail. Let's keep it easy so you and I can actually implement it. When we eat, our digestive system is put into action and it stays active for several hours. If you are like most people, you eat a big meal every 4-5 hours plus snacks. Your digestive system is working all day long and doesn't get a break until you sleep. In fact, some of us snack until bedtime and only sleep for 5-6 hours. Morning comes pretty quick and we start the process all over again. Your body has very little time to ever stop digesting.

By always having nutrients readily available, the body rarely needs to tap into its stored fat for energy. That is one reason why it is hard to lose belly fat and drop pounds in general. It takes the digestive system a full 12 hours from the last meal to clear out the contents, stop digesting, and be in a state of nothingness. When your body has finally tapped out all the easy calories from meals, it will then look to your muscles to break them down for semi-easy energy. It's important to eat enough protein every day so this process doesn't happen. It can be disappointing to realize that even though you lost 15 pounds in two months, you also lost a noticeable difference in your strength. You wanted the fat in your tummy and thighs to disappear but they're still about the same. The next thing your body will break down for energy is stored carbs in the liver. Finally your body is out of the lazy energy and starts breaking down the energy rich fat molecules. Congratulations, your body is now finally eating itself and you are happy to see results on the scale.

After hour 12 of not eating, the body starts to see the most benefits of fasting. This is the point of intermittent fasting, to maximize hours 13-18 of your day. Fasting consistently over time (even just 2x a week) has a positive effect on how insulin is used in your body. The better insulin use, the less likely you will develop diabetes in the future. Nobody wants diabetes. It causes blindness, loss of limbs, and you can't enjoy dessert anymore...how sad is that? There is also evidence that fasting can increase growth hormone levels and increase the release of norepinephrine (both growth hormone and norepinephrine can accelerate fat loss and muscle gain and boost the metabolic rate).

Everyone should continue to exercise during a fasting regimen. Depending on the type of fast you try, I would suggest exercising more on the days that have a full calorie day and rest /recover on the low to no calorie days. If you always eat a full days' worth of calories, exercise during the window of time you eat.

16/8 Fast

also known as Lean Gains® developed by Martain Berkhan

No food or calorie drinks for 16 hours followed by eating your daily calorie goals in the following 8 hours. Many people do this by skipping breakfast because they have already fasted for 7 hours while asleep. It doesn't really matter which meal you decide to skip. Most people have more social obligations in the evening so it makes sense to eat then versus being "that person" who makes everyone else feel awkward because of their personal food choices.

Most of us have a set work schedule that dictates when we eat lunch. If you eat at noon, you can eat until 8 pm, but you won't eat or drink any calories from 8 pm until noon the next day. You may want to drink more water, tea, and coffee if you need something in your belly.

If you take vitamins, wait until you have a meal because most products can upset the stomach if taken on an empty stomach. Always a caveat, if you know the vitamin or supplement should be taken before a meal because your doctor said so, then obviously take those at the correct interval.

I wouldn't beat yourself up if you fail at it in the beginning. Oh no! You only fasted for 14 hours. So what? Great job! Tomorrow is another day to try again. It's always a good idea to break the fast (eat) every day around the same time, but you and I both know that weekends can be crazy. Maybe your family loves having Sunday brunch and you have to cut your fast short. One option is to always plan ahead the day before and eat in a shorter time frame. For example: eat in 6 hours instead of 8 and just deal with that hungry feeling a little longer. If you totally fall off the band wagon one day, just start fresh the next day. Don't beat yourself up about it. This is a guilt-free diet and exercise plan I'm outlining for you.

Again, the 16/8 plan is to not eat (or drink calorie beverages) for 16 hours and only consume your daily calories in an 8-hour window.

24-Hour Fast

    also known as Eat Stop Eat® developed by Brad Pilon

The 24-Hour Fast Method is done twice a week. You eat normally for five days a week and you do not eat (or drink calorie beverages) for two non-consecutive days. A typical week may look like this: You don't eat (or drink calorie beverages) on Tuesday and Thursday and the rest of the week is business as usual.

You can make this easier on yourself by staggering when you start the fast. Personally, I like having something to eat each day so I would eat lunch on Tuesday and then stop eating until Wednesday for dinner. Psychologically, I feel like I can play a mind trick on myself by just causally skipping dinner, having an extra coffee in the morning, and toughing out lunch. At the 24-hour mark, you can either eat a little something or reward yourself with a big dinner to break the fast. You could just as easily skip eating the entire day and not track anything. Just fight it out for 24 hours and use sleep to your advantage. Maybe you can go to bed earlier on those days. Wouldn't it be great to have 9 hours of sleep twice a week?

Alteration: Prepare yourself for the way some people alter this plan. On those 24-hour fast days, some people actually recommend consuming up to 500 calories. That's just enough to cut those headaches and grumpy feelings that may happen when fasting. Maybe try eating a low carb protein shake or an MCT oil coffee so you can sip on it for a longer period of time and feel less like you're fasting and sacrificing.

I think you can handle either of these intermittent fasting options and jumpstart your health goals. Nobody said you have to live this way forever. Perhaps you made a commitment to try one method for two weeks and see how it goes. Maybe you try the other method in the following two weeks and see if you do better. Also keep a journal and write down how you feel throughout the day. Any cravings, annoyances, any other physical or mental things you noticed? Write those down as well. It might be easy for you to tell which method you prefer but if it's hard to tell, then just refer back to the journal and you should be able to find a winner.

Another option is to try one method for two weeks and then no fasting for two weeks. Then switch up the methods. After you read more about the subject, you might absolutely be convinced this is the lifestyle you need to follow. However, the self-discipline required to stick to intermittent fasting for two weeks or longer could be more than you can handle. Maybe you could just do it for one week per month. I think you could, don't you?

29 MAKE THIS SIMPLE CHANGE IN YOUR EXERCISE FOR BETTER RESULTS

Have you ever heard this misguided advice about exercise: *"Don't exercise too hard. Lactic acid will build up and cause a burning sensation in your muscles. Too much of it will ruin your workout."* Well, laboratory science has finally caught up with what I learned in the gym years ago. You need to generate, not avoid, lactic acid during a good workout.

Research by Dr. George Brooks at the University of California, Berkeley showed that your mitochondria (the energy factories in your muscle cells) absorb and use lactic acid as fuel. Lactic acid doesn't stay around long and it has nothing to do with muscle soreness. To make your exercise more effective, focus on gradually increasing the intensity of your workout as you become conditioned. If you are walking, swimming or riding a bicycle, for example, you can time how long it takes you to get to a certain distance and then try to shave five seconds off your time in each of your following workouts at the same distance. In other words, each day you exercise, try to cover the same distance five seconds faster.

This extra challenge shifts you from the aerobic (with oxygen) zone to the anaerobic (without oxygen) zone. By asking your lungs to supply more oxygen than they can handle, you create an oxygen debt, which triggers a series of powerful health-enhancing events. First, you will signal your body to pump up your lung volume - a prime anti-aging tool. Second, you boost the reserve capacity in your heart - critical for avoiding heart attacks. And third, you use lactic acid for fuel, which tells your body to reduce fat building.

Try it out and let me know how it goes!

30 ARE 20 MINUTE WORKOUTS ANY GOOD

I think we both know that exercise is very beneficial to a person's health. So why don't more people exercise on a regular basis? Is it lack of money? Or lack of motivation? Or the lack of equipment? No.

The #1 reason people don't exercise is perceived lack of time.

Martin Gibala, a kinesiology professor and exercise researcher at McMaster University says, "We know that 50% of the population doesn't exercise and the most commonly cited barrier to exercise is the lack of time." Professor Gibala put his theory to the test in a study published in the Journal of Physiology. What he did was compare a group of people who exercised a "traditional" 90 to 120 minutes a day to a group that only exercised 20 minutes a day, and only 3 days a week.

After only two weeks, BOTH groups showed improvement in exercise performance and oxygen uptake. What was interesting is that the improvement was almost identical in both groups. How can that be? They found the group that only exercised for 20 minutes trained with greater focus and intensity. So IT IS possible to get a lot out of short, focused workouts instead of long one-hour workouts. Read the next section to learn more about these intense, interval training workouts.

31 CARDIO HEALTH HACK: INTERVAL TRAINING:

Start (run, elliptical, bicycle etc.) at a normal to slightly less than normal (when first starting) speed for 3 minutes. Then go all out as hard and fast as you can for 20 seconds. Then go back to that normal speed for another 3 minutes. Then go all out again. Keep repeating the pattern, Normal-Fast-Normal, for however long you want, 10-30 minutes. I recommend aiming for 10 minutes to start and only sprint for 20 seconds. Increase that time by ten seconds every 8 days until you are sprinting for a solid 1 minute max. Another way to look at "going max" is to find your max heart rate for your age and body weight online and exercise during that fast time interval at a speed that will increase your heart rate to 75% of that max. There are plenty of products on the market that can measure your heart rate, steps and even products with built-in GPS. I made the mistake of going for a minute on my first try with running and my booty, legs and shins were sore for a solid week. Start slow because I want you to succeed.

Another example: Let's say you only have 20 minutes available for cardio. Before reading this chapter, you would do a 5 speed on a stationary bicycle and when you decided to step it up one day, you would do your allotted time at 8.5 speed. Try this interval training modification. Go at a 12 speed for 1 full minute, drop to a 4.5 speed for 3 minutes and repeat for 20 minutes. You will feel a difference in the exercise intensity and results, guaranteed. By the way, if you are looking for music to get you amped up so you can stay motivated during this intense workout, you can easily find "workout" stations on all the music apps on your phone. RnB, Rap, Dance, Country, Rock all have stations designated as workout, which means the beats per minute are probably at 120 and that translates into a good rhythm to keep pace.

There are dozens of studies that confirm the benefits of shorter but more intense workouts. Just remember that HOW you exercise in those 20 minutes is the important thing. Intensity is the key, not duration. So keep that in mind as you try to get everything into your busy schedule. If you already exercise regularly, then try mixing things up and do a shorter and more intense workout. You'll get a lot out of it and you will save yourself a lot of time.

32 EXERCISES TO HELP YOU REDUCE NECK AND SHOULDER PAIN

As you can probably imagine, I have a lot of patients who struggle with neck and shoulder pain. Many people who work in offices and on computers complain of frequent neck pain and tightness. You may also be a 'looking down' texter and phone user. Here's a way to target the neck and shoulders: dumbbells. Strength training using dumbbells not only reduces pain, but also improves the function of your neck and shoulder area. Here are 5 exercises that you can do with dumbbells to reduce pain and improve function in the neck and shoulders. Just follow the pictures. If you need a long explanation and a better visual aid, search YouTube.

1. The one-arm row

    Get into the position shown. When lifting the weight, don't raise your shoulder to your ear. Keep it in the neutral position as shown and when you raise the weight, make sure you are squeezing the back muscles between your shoulder blades.

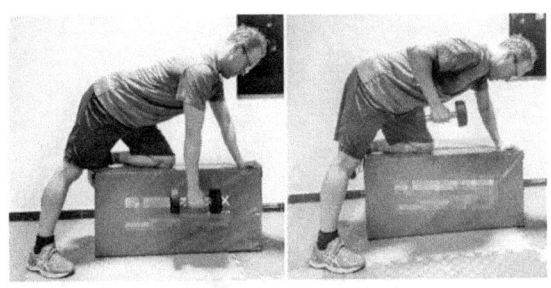

2. Shoulder abduction

   Start in the left picture position. Keep the shoulders down, don't let them raise to your ears. When you raise the arms, the tendency is to try and keep them directly in line with your legs. However, based on how the shoulder joint is angled, I actually have my arms out in front of me at about a 15° angle. You will notice that this slight forward position puts less stress on the shoulder joint on the way up.

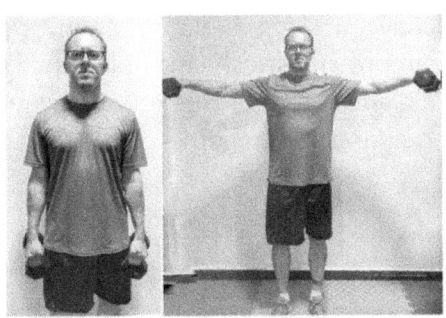

3. Shoulder shrug

   This time, you do want to raise your shoulder to your ear. Do your best to tighten the front and back of the shoulders when lifting. One way to do that is to grip the barbells hard and slightly bend the elbows. You should even feel the biceps and triceps tighten.

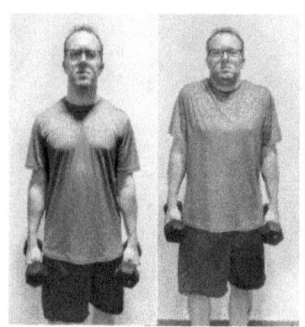

4. Reverse fly

Assume the first picture position. Feet are about shoulder width apart, knees are bent and my chest is a little forward. Notice my back is still straight and not curved. By bending the knees and pushing my butt out, I get this forward position without rounding my back. The weights are not lifted overhead and they are not lifted directly in front of you. Notice, I am lifting the barbells out sideways (elbows have a slight bend so I can grip harder and activate more muscles) and pinching between the shoulder blades. That is the key to this exercise, pinch those shoulder blades together.

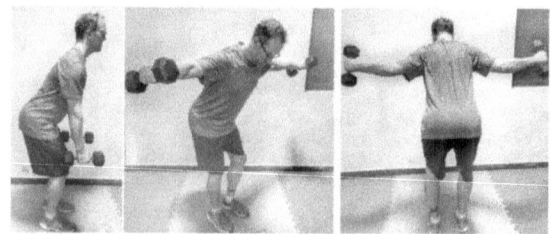

5. Upright row

Keep the shoulders away from your ears on this exercise. When you start raising the weights, bring the hands close together immediately and raise to your collar bone.

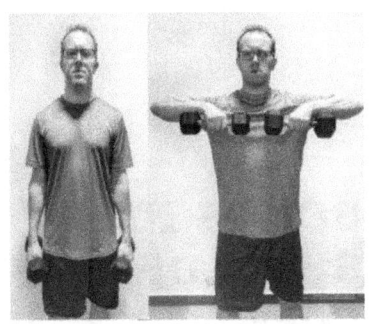

Start with light hand weights of about 4-12 pounds. Perform these exercises 3 times per week and mix up your workouts if you don't want to do all 5 each time. One routine could be to do exercises 1, 2, and 5 one day, and then exercises 1, 3, and 4 the next. Switch back and forth each time you exercise. When starting out, do each motion 10-12 times and repeat that twice. As you get stronger, add a third set. Once you can do an exercise comfortably for 3 sets, increase the weight by 2-3 pounds. Focus on technique and try to go up/down or in/out (depending on the exercise) for a count of 4 seconds each way. This means: take 4 seconds to bring the arm all the way up and take 4 seconds to bring it all the way down.

33 BONUS IDEA FOR THE SHOULDER - ROTATOR CUFF

When I do my shoulder rotator cuff workout, I keep it to very light weights. My profession requires a lot of shoulder motions and I want those little shoulder muscles to be strong and high endurance. I do the above exercises but I add internal-external rotation with my arm and elbow by my side, followed by the arm and elbow lifted to 90° for 10 reps with 5-8 pound weights. My goal is not to engage the bigger muscle groups but to focus solely on the small, weaker, stabilizing rotator cuff area.

People tend to ignore the small muscles and always want to put more and more weight on their bench and shoulder press. They tend to sacrifice good technique and are prone to have overuse injuries of the shoulder. This means they tend to develop a deep ache in the shoulder joint and will experience pain with a normal range of motion, but especially when stressing it with weight lifting. If they would just back off the weight a few days a week, focus on perfect technique and go slow, they would notice that the joint and tendons heal. Also, as I mentioned, they could focus on really light weights and work on the unsexy muscles like the rotator cuff and deep hip/gluteus muscles because these muscles stabilize and strengthen the pivotal joints. What they would find out after a month of focusing on these stabilizing muscles is that when they do lift heavy weights, their technique will be improved, more power will be generated, and more weight can be lifted.

34 3 EASY EXERCISES TO TONE YOUR STOMACH

A lot of my patients exercise and one thing that is becoming more popular is "core training." Core training is exercising the "core" of your body, which many think of as your abs. Truth be told, the core is way more than just the abs. If all you did were crunches and sit-ups, you would be missing two-thirds of the core. The most complete core package will also target the sides of your stomach/abdomen as well as your deep back spinal muscles. The sides of your stomach have muscles that run left and right as well as at an angle. They act like a corset when they contract and if you make these strong, it just sucks your whole abdomen in more. Talk about making your abs look great and have your self-esteem jump up a notch. I'm here to tell you one more reason, besides vanity, to make your core strong.

Many back disorders and leg soreness stems from the abs, back, front and back pelvis and legs all being out of muscular sync. If your abs are weak then your back muscles over contract and over load the spine; if your front pelvis muscles are to strong (to many sit-ups) then it can cause the spine to have too much curve and again over load the discs; and finally, your gluts (butt) and hamstrings (back leg muscles) can be weak causing your pelvis to tilt forward and again pain occurs. Make it a habit to get all three areas strong because not only does it look and feel good but a tight core will help your body age well and will set you up for good posture and a pain-free lower back.

Having a slim stomach area takes more than exercise. You probably know that it also takes cardiovascular exercise and a proper diet. In fact, if you want to see your abs then you have to be less than 10% body fat. Guess what? Eating a lot of carbs and dairy and not being strict with your diet will always lead to hidden abs, regardless of how big you make them. However, these are two killer moves you can do at home to strengthen all 3 core muscle groups at once. Now that's efficient.

Exercise #1: The Plank

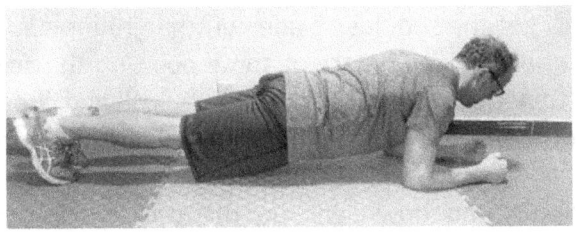

Start out in a push up position on the floor but place your weight on the forearms not the hands. Keep your forearms in place like the picture. To start in a neutral position, just bring the knees to the ground. When you are ready, raise your chest, pelvis and knees so they are all off the ground in a flat line (like the picture). Notice the pelvis is level with the back and not poking up higher causing an upside down V shape. Tighten your abdominal muscles, shoulders and your butt muscles and hold this position for 20 seconds. Rest for 15 seconds and repeat up to 3 times. After a few days, add 10 seconds and continue adding until you can hold the position for 60 seconds without shaking. Do this 5 times a week.

Exercise #2: Butterfly Abs

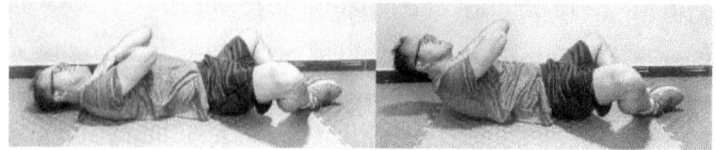

Sit on the floor with the soles of your feet touching, so your knees flare out like the picture. Now lie back on the floor and try to tilt your pelvis so that the lower back is in contact with the floor too. Typically when we lay back, our lumbar (low back) will be arched and not touching. Now cross your arms over your chest, contract your abs and raise your chest so that the shoulder blades are off the ground about 4 inches. Be mindful to actually get the shoulder blades off the ground and not just bend the neck. I like to stare at some point on the ceiling and raise up to get closer to it. This way, the neck and chest stay in alignment, therefore avoiding neck pain. Look at the picture, I did NOT do a sit up but I did do about ½ of a crunch. Those 4 inches of up and down will do the trick while minimizing unwanted injuries. Do 20 reps, rest, do 20 more and do this 5 times a week.

35 BONUS EXERCISE: SUCKING IN THE GUT VERSUS HOLLOWING THE ABDOMINALS

I'm talking to the obvious crowd here, guys who have a belly but realize they can suck it in and hide that extra girth. You know the scene: walking around town, pretty girl is in sight, you instinctively suck your belly in, the shirt stops poking out and you think, "yeah, this girl finds me attractive." Hold the laughter because I have a point to make. Instead of sucking your belly in, there is actually a movement you can do that exercises your core more and if done regularly will make a difference in strength for you, and still have the same thinning effect. A little known fact: sucking the belly in can actually weaken the abs a bit.

Let me tell you about Abdominal Hollowing. If I were about to punch you in the stomach, you would do a full core tightening so that when I strike you, it wouldn't hurt so much. Go ahead, have your friend punch you in the stomach, I'll wait. Ok, see how you contracted to dull the blow? You can teach yourself how to walk around like that. (Another example is the way we tighten our core when you try to void your bowels with a constipation feeling in the restroom).

Step 1: Tilt the pelvis forward and up and hold it here. The motion is like trying to have your front lower pelvis (the pubic bone, the bone above your genitals) and belly button touch each other or at least bring them closer together. It's a similar motion you see when a dancer is thrusting their pelvis back and forth, up and down and their booty jiggles.

Step 2: You have your pelvis tilted; now contract your abs, like you did before you got punched.

Step 3: Practice breathing in this contracted state. As an exercise, you can hold this position for a count of 10 to begin with. If you want to increase the time to 30 seconds, then it is essential that you learn to breathe while contracting.

Once you master this, it's time to show off your "flat belly" at the supermarket any time you want and get a little exercise to boot.

36 EXERCISES TO HELP STRENGTHEN THE LOW BACK AND THE UNKNOWN CORE MUSCLES

When you look at the exercises I have laid out for you, one of the thoughts that cross your mind could be: That is just too easy. Or maybe: No way will these basic exercises will do anything for me. My only reply is, humbly, you are wrong. Let me explain.

I worked in China for one year and then moved back to the good ol' USA. Ten months later, my old China hospital CEO opens a dialogue about wanting me back. This time around, he wants me there for a longer period of time and to eventually start integrating full-blown exercise routines for the patients. When I was in Colorado, I had an awesome computer program that had 2-3 types of stretches, ball exercises and three different levels of exercise difficulty including dumbbells as a 4th level. I combed through all the options and created three stages of rehab for each body part that I treat. One day, my work PC just wasn't cutting it, so I upgraded to the latest version, reinstalled the programs I needed then found out that the program would not install on anything but XP. To this day, they still have not updated it even though the website says they will. Being a smart guy, I made a master copy, put it in a box with a few other important things for safe keeping, and somehow managed to lose that box when I moved to Louisiana. I'll take a pity party please. Therefore, I recreated what I could for my clinic in Louisiana and narrowed a lot of things down to what is absolutely necessary. I found myself only highlighting one third of a packet in Colorado for people to actually perform anyway. Once I decided to return to China, I wanted to be prepared for implementing exercises immediately. I work with a translator and not everyone speaks real Mandarin, so even the translator needs a translator for many people. Plus, many are farmers and never have been exposed to real stretching and exercises like most of us Americans have. This means I needed to keep what I show them easy to explain, easy to perform, not overwhelm them with 15 exercises and have maximum benefit for all their disc bulges and muscle pain. I spent a considerable amount of time researching what exercises could be given for a large variety of conditions without causing them more issues, and what has been shown and proven in the research to be real winners. The following four exercises are what I came up with. The official program hasn't started in that hospital so these are what I give as a general "you need to do some kind of active rehab to stabilize and strengthen the injured area."

Bird Dog:

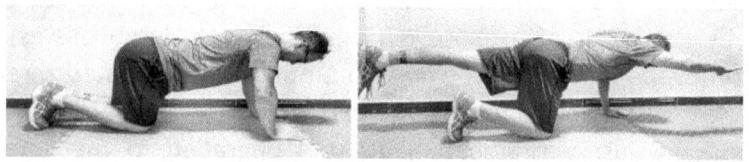

Start out on all fours. Notice that the elbows are bent 10-15 so that the shoulders can be at the same level as your butt. Bring one leg straight out and raise it level with your butt. It's common to over lift it so the pelvis will look higher on that side. Check yourself in a mirror to make sure it is level. Next raise the opposite arm and keep your neck in a straight (neutral) position. The opposite elbow is still bent because the shoulders need to be level; if you over raise your arm, it will mean your shoulders are no longer level. Be sure to contract your abs and your butt. Hold for 30 seconds on each side and repeat 3 times. Do this 4 times per week.

Plank:

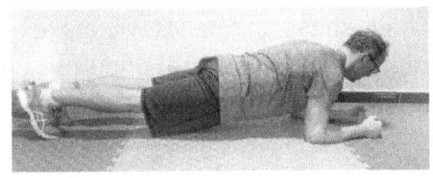

Start out in a push up position on the floor but place your weight on the forearms not the hands. Keep your forearms in place like the picture. To start in a neutral position, just bring the knees to the ground. When you are ready, raise your chest, pelvis and knees so they are all off the ground in a flat line (like the picture). Notice the pelvis is level with the back and not poking up higher causing an upside down V shape. Tighten your abdominal muscles and your butt muscles and hold this position for 20 seconds. Rest for 15 seconds and repeat up to 3 times. After a few days, add 10 seconds and continue adding until you can hold the position for 60 seconds without shaking. Do this 5 times a week.

Side Plank:

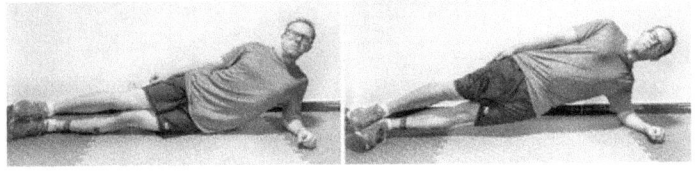

Start on your side with the elbow and forearm on the ground holding your torso up. The elbow needs to be aligned under the shoulder for stability on the next step. Stack your feet on top of each other. Next, lift your pelvis and knees off the ground, supporting your weight on the arm. Be sure to contract your abdominal and gluteus areas and make a strong shoulder contraction. Those who are untrained in this motion will see their back and arm start shaking in 12 seconds. Do your best and try and hold for 30 seconds on each side and repeat 3 times. Do this 4 times per week. If you just can't do it, then bend the knees 90 (your feet, knees and pelvis will make an L shape with the feet pointed directly behind you) and raise up on the knees instead of the feet.

Hip Bridge:

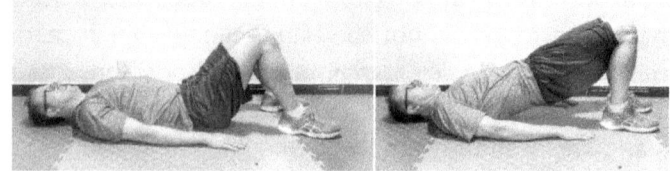

Start with your back on the ground, knees bent, feet shoulder width apart and arms to the side. Use your abs and butt to raise your pelvis off the floor. You want the chest and pelvis to be level. The best way to cheat is to use your leg muscles to raise and keep you at this level position. That's cheating, so don't do it, just contract your core. Hold for 30 seconds on each side and repeat 3 times. Do this 4 times per week. Too easy? Kick a foot out so one leg is fully straight. Alternate sides.

37 A QUICK AND EASY STRETCH FOR BACK PAIN SUFFERERS AND DESK WORKERS

A lot of my patients get lower back pain and/or stiffness due to sitting for long periods of time. Whether it's sitting at your desk or working on your computer, long drives in the car, long airline trips, or even bleacher seats at ball games, sitting can trigger back pain, especially as we get older. Did you know that 80-90% of all Americans will experience back pain in their lives? It's true! In addition to chiropractic adjustments, stretching the right muscles is one of the best ways to avoid chronic back pain, especially if you have trouble sitting for a long period of time.

The bottom line is that we lose flexibility as we age. And if we don't stretch, our flexibility will be even worse. If you sit at a desk all day, you make things even worse for your back pain. The front pelvis muscles get tight, short and pull on the spine causing discomfort. Therefore, it is important to keep the correct spinal stabilizing muscles strong and flexible. The added benefit of the exercises presented in this book, as well as the current Runner's Stance stretch, will be a reduction in pain.

I want to show you a quick and easy stretch for low back pain that will benefit you. What you want to do is stretch the front of your hips and legs either daily or every other day. This area of your body is called your hip flexors. If you sit all day, you put a lot of pressure and stress on your hip flexors. And if your hip flexors get tight and stiff, it will lead to low back pain. If you sit for long periods of time each day, you should find this stretch very beneficial.

What you want to do is stand with your left foot forward and your right foot back, with your feet flat on the floor. Then, either put your hands on your hips or have a chair next to you that you can hold on to for support. Make sure you keep your back and hips in straight alignment. Next, push your hips forward while keeping your back leg straight. If you notice the left knee is further than your foot, then you need to bring your foot farther out in front of you. The knee should stay even with the ankle (not drifting forward over the foot and toes), otherwise you run a risk of injuring the knee. Slowly, keep moving your hips forward until you feel a comfortable level of tension in your legs and front hip. If you find yourself really low to the ground and think this exercise is a joke, raise up a little and then bring your chest back. It's highly likely your chest and back are bent over instead of in a neutral upright position. Hold for 10 to 15 seconds. Then switch sides and do the other leg. Do each side 3 times.

- I recommend getting out of you chair and walking around every 55 minutes.
- I recommend doing this stretch at mid-morning and mid-afternoon while at work.

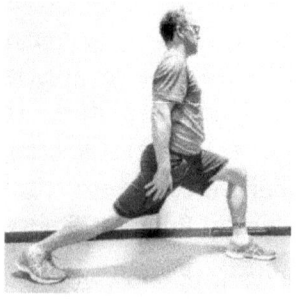

38 WHEN SHOULD I STRETCH?

Tip 1: In general, I never recommend stretching your muscles before you exercise, when your muscles are 'cold.' Research has shown not only is it worthless to stretch before your muscles are warm and full of blood, it can also lead to injury. With that note, do 5 minutes of cardio or fast walking to get the blood circulating and then do a light stretch. My biggest recommendation, and one that finally helped me recover from a pulled groin, is to take 5 minutes and go through a variety of stretches after your workout. Think of your warm muscles like hot gelatin. If I can mold hot gelatin into any shape I want as it cools, then I want my hot gelatin legs and other muscles to cool off in a nice elongated shape.

Tip 2: A nice way to stretch for long-term physical gains.

In the morning, pick two stretches and hold them each for 30 seconds. Wait two hours then do those same two stretches for 30 seconds again. In another 2 hours, do those same two again for 20 seconds. This technique will allow you to keep the stretch gains you made, otherwise the muscles tend to just tighten up again.

Tip 3: Don't bend the first 20 minutes in the morning.

Throughout the night, the lumbar discs have had time to plumb up and if you already have disc issues, bending over can stress the bulge and cause a flare up. Another reason is that the tendons, ligaments and other surrounding tissues have had time to shorten and tighten up and a sudden stretch on them could cause an injury. Think of a fresh cut that has a bandage on it: after a few hours when you take the bandage off, fresh skin gets ripped off too. I'm sure you heard of someone picking up a pair of socks on the floor and then their back goes out. Well, I'm 100% sure that the weight of the sock that morning wasn't the real cause of the disc injury and subsequent back pain.

39 WHAT ARE NERVE GLIDE/ FLOSSING STRETCHES AND HOW THEY STOP NUMBNESS IN THE ARMS AND LEGS

Basics of how nerves travel in the body and why they can get injured

Numbness and tingling can occur in any part of your arm or leg. Nerves branch out of your spinal cord and pass through holes in your spine. The nerves that come out of the last few neck vertebrae will travel to different parts of your arm. Your thumb and second finger, 3rd finger, and 4-5th finger are supplied by different nerves; this is why you may only feel tingling in two fingers and not the whole hand. The nerves that come out of the last few low back vertebrae travel down your leg; it's the back of your leg and buttock where you normally start to feel the tingling sensations. Again, which the side of your calf, back of your leg, or part of the foot is numb will let the doctor know which nerves are truly the issue.

Muscles and ligaments can be injured for all types of reasons: sports, sitting too long, car accidents, etc. When these tissues heal, they are never quite the same. I'm sure you have a scar somewhere on your body, which is proof that the body can heal itself, but it heals with different, less optimal tissue. When an injury is healed with scar tissue or if a muscle is overly tight where the nerves pass, that can lead to numbness and tingling.

Think of the nerves like a rope anchored to the spine and passing down the arm or leg next to muscles and bones. The rope has only a certain amount of space to move freely and every time your limb moves, that nerve/ rope is expected to stretch, glide, and shift with no resistance.

Continuing the illustration, what happens when any rope is placed between two heavy bricks and you try to pull the rope through? You feel resistance. Can the rope pass through the bricks? Sure, but it takes more effort and the rope would fray over time. That is a good way to think about a nerve being trapped by two overly tight muscles. It cannot move freely, pressure builds up on certain areas of the nerve, and the fibers can become irritated and cause numbness downstream.

What happens when a rope rests on the edge of a metal box with a heavy brick on top of it and you are trying to pass the rope though it? You encounter the same issue as before but now that rope will become frayed. When a nerve gets frayed from being sandwiched between muscles and bone, this obviously creates pain and numbness, and swelling of the nerve and the tissues around it. Neither scenario is ideal for a nerve. A nerve likes to move freely and not get hung up by scar tissue, adhesions, tight muscles, or anything else.

What are Adhesions?

You could have arthritis in the spine, overly tight muscles, old injuries that have scar tissue and/ or bulges. Yes, you could have all four at the same time. Because of all the different reasons you can have numbness and tingling, it's a good idea to get checked out by a chiropractor, physical therapist, or a medical doctor. Let's assume you have been checked and no cancer, tumors, or other serious red flag is present. Now, let's assume you have been getting some rehab and a round of adjustments and your pain is mostly gone but a little bit of numbness is dragging on and nagging you. You could almost go back to your daily life like normal but you still get numbness and shooting pain when you perform certain motions specific to your lifestyle and job requirements.

It's quite possible that the nerves have formed some pesky connections to muscles and ligaments that shouldn't normally be there. These ill-placed connections are called adhesions and they could be the culprit to your numbness and tingling. Let's illustrate with an example: you are watering your flowers and are dragging the hose. Everything is great until you round the corner and the hose brushes up to a highly textured bark of a tree. Now when you walk farther, you notice the hose "catching" and rubbing and you either have to drag it harder and risk tearing the hose (or the tree) or walk over to the tree and move the hose. We both know the second option is best. The hose "catching" on the bush causing you resistance when you drag the hose is similar to the nerve "catching" on the adhesions of muscles.

What are Nerve Flossing Stretches?

I think you see why you might be experiencing the numbness and tingling in your arms and legs now. You are now ready to do some self-guided stretches called Neuro-Flossing. The following pages will walk you through specific science-based stretches that are clinically shown to break up those adhesions and allow the nerves to move and glide freely again. Do you want that? Would you like those nerves to heal and get back to your normal life? I know you do.

I did my best to explain how to do each stretch and also show a picture or two for each to clear up any confusion. When I give these to patients, the explanations are much less detailed because I walk them through each and the picture along with a simple explanation should act as a trigger for them to remember how to do it.

You can do it. **If you feel extra pain or a little too much of that "stretch" feeling, please back off. These are NERVE stretches (not muscles), so a little stretch goes a long way. Stay pain free with these. DO NOT GET AGGRESSIVE.**

* Regardless of which nerve is the issue in the neck, do all the neck neuro-flossing stretches.

Low Back and Leg Numbness & Tingling

Stretch for Disc Bulges

Start with your face and chest flat on the ground. Then raise your chest so your back arches and lean your head back. Keep the pelvis on the floor. Try to straighten out your arms. Hold for 15 seconds. Repeat 3 times. Do this twice a day, 4 times a week

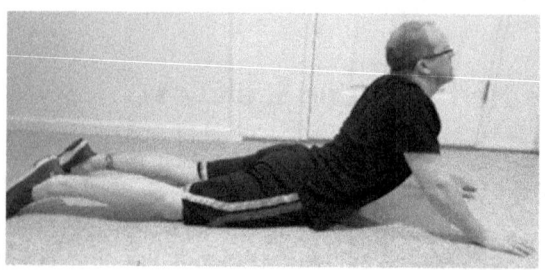

Sciatic Nerve

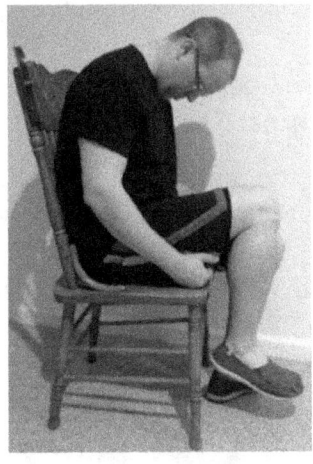

Part 1: (left picture) Sit with the affected leg slightly elevated off chair and in a bent knee position with the foot pointed down. The head should be looking down at your chest and slump *your chest forward.*

Part 2: (right picture) Straighten out the leg and point the foot toward you. The chest should now be arched backward (or at least straight) and the head tilted backwards.

Hold each position for 5 seconds and repeat 5 times. Do this 2 times a day for 4 days a week.

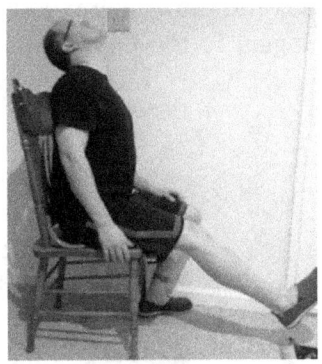

Neck and Arm and Hand Numbness & Tingling

Start Here: Top 3 Stretches

Do all of these twice a day and 4 times a week.
Hold each position for 5 seconds and repeat 5 times

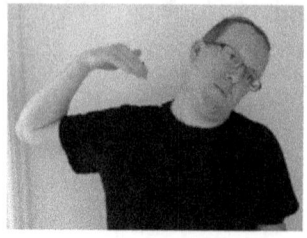

1a. Raise the affected arm 90°, even with the shoulder. Bend the elbow 45° and point your hand, fingers and wrist (loosely) toward your ear. Bend your head away from that hand.

1b. Straighten out your arm with the palm facing up and now point your fingers to the floor. Bend your head toward that hand.

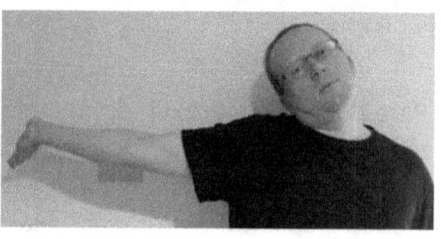

2. (Left) Keep the arm straight (don't bend the elbow) and bring the arm backwards with the palm up (like grabbing a baton) and turn your head to look at your hand. Only do one arm at a time.

3. (Right) Hands up, arms bent 90°, and raise the elbows all the way so they're even with the

top of the shoulders. Pinch the shoulders backward, bringing the shoulder blades together. Keep your head even and try to glide the head backwards so that your ears are over your shoulder (look at the picture on 5 for the neck/head position).

Median Nerve

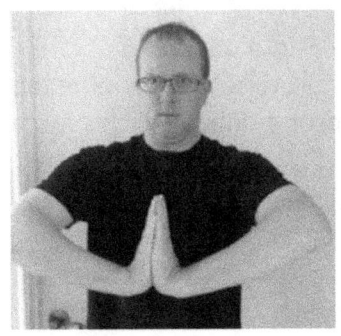

Start with both **palms** touching each other with the arms out in front of you near the chest muscles. Keep elbows level and bring your **wrists/hands down**. Lower your hands as if trying to get to the belly button. Stop lowering once the bottom of your palms start to separate. Hold it right there for 5 seconds.

Repeat 5 times. Do this twice a day and 4 times a week.

Regardless of which nerves are causing the issue in the neck, do all the neck neuro-flossing stretches.

Radial Nerve

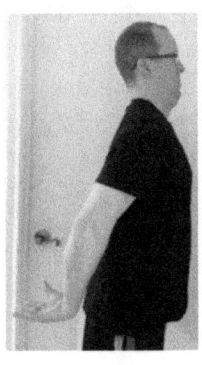

5. Tuck and pull your chin backwards So you have a 'double' chin. Keep the arm straight (don't bend the elbow) and bring the arm backwards with the palm up (like grabbing a baton).

Only do one arm at a time. Hold it for 5 seconds, Repeat 5 times. Do this twice a day and 4 times a week.

6. Start with the **back of the hands** (near the wrist) touching each other with the arms out in front of you. Keep elbows level and bring your **wrists/hands up**. (The wrists start at your chest, raise them towards the ceiling.) Stop raising once the wrists start to separate on the top. Hold it right there for 5 seconds. Repeat 4 times.. Do this twice a day and 4 times a week.

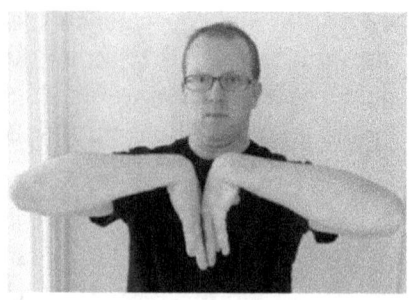

Regardless of which nerves are causing the issue in the neck, do all the neck neuro-flossing stretches.

Ulnar Nerve

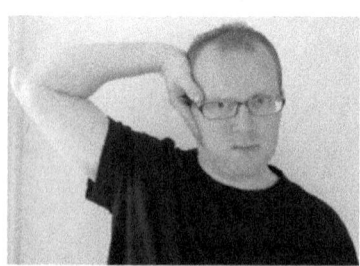

Do one arm at a time.
Cup your ear with your fingers pointing up and then rotate your hand backwards so the fingers point to the back of your head; the finishing point is when the fingers are pointing down like in the picture. Try and position your wrist on top of the ear. This requires some flexibility so at least aim for the temple.
Hold for 10 seconds. Repeat 4 times. Do this twice a day, 4 times a week.

40 BONUS: 6 WAYS TO ELIMINATE HEADACHES BEFORE THEY START

With all the stress going on these days, I've noticed a lot of people complaining about headaches. So I wanted to give you:

5 ways you can eliminate headaches before they even start... WITHOUT pills!

=====================
1. Obey Your Alarm Clock
=====================

According to Dr. Lisa Mannix, a spokeswoman for the National Headache Foundation in Chicago, pressing your snooze button may turn you into a head case. As it turns out, snoozing for more than an hour after the alarm clock goes off can disrupt your sleep-wake cycle and set you up for a tension headache later in the day.

==========
2. Eat Smart
==========

The substances in processed food--such as nitrates in luncheon meat and monosodium glutamate (MSG) in some ready-to-eat food items--can trigger a migraine in certain people. To be certain that you don't get "hit in the head" when you least expect it, grab an easy-to-eat fruit or almonds when you feel hungry. Better yet, make an effort to lessen your consumption of processed food.

=============
3. Get Adjusted
=============

In her article, "Stop a Headache Before It Starts," Jaydine Sayer explains: "The main sensory nerve in your forehead is rooted at the base of your neck--which is why experiencing muscle tension there or in your shoulders can lead to head pain." When the spinal bones in the neck get locked up and subluxated, it will cause muscle tension and nerve irritation that can cause headaches. Getting chiropractic adjustments regularly easily solves this problem for most people.

============
4. Drink Water
============

Doctors reveal that dehydration is a common cause of headaches. When your body loses fluids, you also begin to "wilt" like a parched plant. All your body functions go haywire and pretty soon you'll feel your head throbbing. It's worth repeating: half your body weight and drink that volume of water in ounces. If you drink tea or coffee, add that same amount of water back into your daily quota. Yes, you will urinate a lot the first few days if you aren't used to it, but your kidneys will balance out.

5. Take a Breather

Tension headaches set in when you're stressed out. This is when your cortisol and adrenaline levels surge. When this happens, your body is forced to pump out sugar. "The rapid change in glucose levels can set you up for pain. You have to give yourself a few minutes to decompress so stress won't get to you," states Sayer. Find what works for you to relax: a bubble bath, walk in the park, music, exercise, focusing on your breath etc.

6. Use a Foam Curve Pillow

I recommend using a foam pillow with a curve or hump in it. Typically, the pillow will have a big and small hump. They also come in different materials so pick one that you like and are not allergic to. Most of these pillows come in a thin, medium, and thick version. If you are a back sleeper then you probably only need the thin. Side sleepers need to measure the distance between their ear and the edge of their shoulder on an imaginary horizontal line from the ear. If you use a ruler, one side of the ruler is touching your ear and the other side is not touching anything. A pillow should be a similar size to that measurement. Too small or too thick and your neck will be in a sustained overstretched position, which will lead to headaches and stiffness. I would lean towards a thinner size if you can't find one that is just right. It might take a few nights to get used to the new pillow. Always buy one with a 30-day warranty as you might have to try several different materials or brands to find your perfect sleeping tool.

41 HIDDEN ERGONOMIC TIP: STOP THE 3PM HEADACHE?

The neck and shoulder routine is obviously basic and is meant more for the person who is starting from scratch. It can also be appropriate for those who have pain in their neck or shoulders or had an injury recently and want to do something for self-care. Truth be told, someone could do these to strengthen that area so they don't get pain to begin with.

Headaches experienced in the afternoon could be from overworked neck muscles while using a computer. Doing these exercises will build endurance in these supporting neck muscles and hopefully stop the muscles from fatiguing and getting headaches in the first place. I would recommend raising your computer screen to where your eyes are at mid-screen level. This may mean bringing those worthless thick phone books to work and stacking them so the screen is higher.

42 BONUS: STUDY SHOWS LOST SLEEP CANNOT BE MADE UP

If you think staying in bed on the weekends will make up for a week's worth of sleep deprivation, think again. A new study finds that going long periods without sleep can lead to a sort of "sleep debt" that cannot simply be undone with a little extra snoozing from time to time. However, the study involved a small number of participants, so further research would be needed to verify the results. Such chronic sleep loss may eventually interfere with your performance on tasks that require focus, becoming particularly noticeable at nighttime when the body's natural sleep-wake cycle isn't giving you an extra boost.

Anyone who's ever pulled an all-nighter knows how debilitating sleep loss can be in the short term. Indeed, studies show that after 24 hours without sleep, a person's performance can drop to the level of someone who is legally drunk. But what if those all-nighters turned into all-weekers? The authors of the current study turned their attention to long-term sleep loss and examined whether the effects of such constant sleep deprivation could be erased with an extended resting period. The researchers put nine young adults on a sleep schedule that a doctor or medical resident might experience on an on-call shift --about 33 hours spent awake followed by 10 hours sleeping; a cycle that is equivalent to about 5.6 hours of sleep every 24 hours. The participants continued on this grueling schedule for three weeks, at which time they were considered chronically sleep deprived. The study also had a control group of eight young adults who were not sleep deprived. The subjects needed to periodically complete a performance task designed to test their ability to pay attention and their reaction time. The sleep-deprived subjects generally performed the same as those who had sufficient sleep if the test was given early on in the day; just two hours after the subjects had awakened from their long rest. This finding held true across all three weeks of the study, suggesting that a long period of shut-eye could temporarily make up for the chronic sleep loss.

However, the subjects performed significantly worse on tests that were given later in the day; after 30 hours spent awake, as the study progressed in weeks. For instance, the subjects fared poorly on the last test of the day they took during week three as compared with that same test during week 1. While they had a median reaction time of 667 milliseconds in testing during week 1, this increased to 2,013 milliseconds by week 3. The subjects appeared to have developed a sleep debt -- all that lost sleep really was catching up with them.

Here's how the results might play out in the real world: An individual who is constantly sleep deprived during weekdays might try to catch up during weekends. While that individual might feel recovered after their sleeping spell, the study suggests the next time they try to go without shut-eye their performance may start to deteriorate. The findings also suggest that short-term and long-term sleep loss may actually act on the brain in two different ways. The sleep debt was also found to be most noticeable during the subject's nighttime. This could be due to the effects of our natural sleep-wake cycle, or circadian rhythm, the researchers suggest. This cycle goes hand-in-hand with the periods of light/dark we experience as the sun rises and sets. Our natural tendency to be awake during the day may mask signs of sleep debt when it's light out. But this protective effect may go away as darkness arrives, the researchers say.

The findings are particularly applicable to people who work odd-hour jobs that may mean they go without sleep for extended periods, such as health workers, truckers and emergency responders. Chronic sleep loss could leave these individuals "vulnerable to accidents and errors," researchers say. They advise public health campaigns to emphasize the "potentially covert consequences of chronic sleep loss." The study was conducted by Daniel Cohen, of Brigham and Women's Hospital in Boston, Mass., and colleagues. The findings were published in the Jan. 13 issue of the Journal of Science Translational Medicine. So if you aren't getting enough sleep, it's important to understand the consequences. Try to get a normal night's sleep as often as you can so that your body doesn't slowly break down.

43 MAKING A BUDGET

How often do you stress out about finances? Does it keep you up at night or delay you actually falling asleep when you rest your head on your pillow? I do hope it's a comfortable foam type with a neck curve in it (Chapter 40). Would your spouse say you have a short temper and are hard to be around when the money gets short at the end of your pay period? Do you fight regularly about that cup of coffee, new pair of shoes, eating out, or getting a drink with friends? You are not alone.

I get it and I've been there myself before. I lived on a tight budget for most of my adult life: being an undergrad and then going to chiropractic college and starting a new clinic. Before going into what I learned from those times in my life, let's back up to my childhood foundations. An important lesson my parents instilled in me was the value of money and how to save for things you want and need.

If you guessed they gave me an allowance then you would be correct. The allowance was something like $1-2 a week. I remember saving up for a month or more and getting a really complicated airplane-based Transformer® toy. It was purple, looked like a fighter jet, and my dad had to help me transform it the first time. Another fond memory was a little older in life when Nintendo 64 was all the rage. Again, I saved for a while and then we drove to the video game store and I rented a hockey game. Half an hour into playing, I get a call from my best friend inviting me for a sleep over. I was torn on because I couldn't bring the game since he didn't have that system. My dad told me to make a decision and live with the results...or something like that. Looking back, that was a great lesson on choices and consequences of actions. I choose to leave and my younger brother was able to play it without me giving him a hard time. Win-win I suppose.

Not everyone has had the luxury of an allowance. Regardless of your past and what you may have been taught or not and any of the mistakes you have made in your life up until now, you can change. You can change not only for your own benefit, but if you have children, you can now help them tackle one of the biggest challenges in life: a budget.

Hang with me a moment and I will discuss my adult life's, dare I admit, cheapness. During undergraduate studies, my family helped me out so I didn't have a job to distract me from studying. I had to find a way to eat and be entertained on about $350 a month. They did cover room and board in the dorms and what a great experience in life that was, so thank you, parents.

I went to the cafeteria to eat one meal a day, typically dinner, because it was buffet style every day. If you ever wondered why freshmen gain 15 pounds, it's because we have an endless supply of pizza, hamburgers, juice, etc., three times a day. Lunch was typically at the student union because it was most convenient between classes. The union had fast food type restaurants, much like you find at a mall food court. I didn't buy the full value meal (no drink and no fries or side dish) because I would run out of money before the end of the month. Peanut butter and jelly sandwiches were a staple of my lunch diet as well. I had one of those small dorm size fridges and breakfast came out of there as well as any leftovers from eating out and meals my mom sent me back to college with after a visit. Sure, when I did go home, she did four loads of laundry and sent me back with four days worth of dinner, but I never said she didn't spoil me.

Another reason to budget and pinch all my pennies was the hope of asking a girl out and be able to pay for it. I couldn't very well give her option A or B and ignore the rest of the menu because I was poor. I know that's hard to believe a lady wouldn't sign up for date two after I recommended the side salad and soup.

Life demanded I have a budget and get creative so I could have a social life and not experience hunger pains or, worse, ask for more money. Many of my closest friends belonged to a Christian organization that met at a building right off campus. This place was fantastic. There was a full-size indoor basketball court, removable volleyball net, TV, couches, showers, full kitchen, and people would show up all the time to hang out and study. The building became a great place to invite people to as well as just visiting with friends. Since it was a ministry to college kids, all the events planned were geared for low cost, maximum fun. You can't beat the comradery and connections that were forged from this group. They had one big problem, however. After an event ended around 10 pm, we were young and didn't want to go home. Many times our after party would be a late night restaurant, and all of a sudden I spent $20 multiple times a week. Add those costs to football games and normal fun activities and you can run into a budget crisis before the last week of the month. Unless I enjoyed eating PB&J twice a day for a week, I had to figure a way to skip those restaurants, maybe get coffee at $3 instead, stretch my budget, and still enjoy socializing.

Chiropractic college wasn't much different. I got into massive debt. With the cost of tuition and books three times a year, a basic apartment, the hours in class and outside to actually learn the material; I would say less than 5% of people even had a part-time job much less anything that could cover all the expense. The solution to most people in all types of post graduate education (dentists, medical doctors, Ph.D. candidates) is to get student loans to cover tuition and living expenses. Here's why I stayed cheap. Every dollar I spend had to be paid back, plus interest. I already took the money as a loan so if I spent it on something frivolous like a new car because the bank account was full or I was eating out several times a week, I owed even more.

One thing that these student loan companies are dishonest about is your potential for more debt after graduation. They make it sound like all this student loan debt is in a special category that doesn't factor in or at least isn't weighed as heavily as debts like cars, credit cards, and boats when the bank analyzes your debt to income ratios. Why is this important?

When we finish school, chiropractors tend to have one of two options. You can work for another doctor or you can open up your own clinic. Opening a clinic requires lots of capital, a fancy word for money. You find the perfect location with the right car traffic, house income, chiropractor to population ratio, and all is right in the world. Now you realize that rent is X amount and that the tenant is responsible to build the walls, the floors, decorate, furnish, buy equipment etc. and all this is way more money than you accounted for.

After 15 different bank loan applications, they all say the same thing, "Sir you have a six-figure debt and you have zero experience running a business much less a profitable one and you have close to zero collateral. You are just too much risk for this bank and we can't loan you the money."

Luckily for me, I had classmates who were second generation chiropractic students and were forewarned about some of these realities. My plan was to be cheap, save up as much of that student loan money as I could, and hopefully have enough cash saved to open on my own clinic and show the banks I had collateral or at least some skin in the game. NEWS FLASH- it didn't help and I was denied left and right.

Eating PB&J in the car while driving to the restaurant just to enjoy the conversation, not buying nicer clothes for the clinic, and renting movies on RedBox didn't amount to anything for the banks.

Fast forward to post graduation and I persevered with my low cost living and was able to show family members I had enough saved and was motivated and courageous enough for them to loan me the difference to purchase a clinic. Next thing you know, I'm a proud owner of an established clinic that was seeing a rapid decline in every measurable area of a business, despite being creatively positioned with misleading statistics when making the purchase. Bamboozled is a nice way to say it. In all fairness, my business coach was cautious about the numbers and warned me about what was probably going on. He still advised I purchase it because once you factor in all the build out and equipment purchases, you spend roughly the same amount; at least by purchasing an existing clinic, you have a list of names you can entice to return and patients still actively getting treatment.

Little did I know just how much wheeling and dealing, special deals, and professional courtesy discounts were being given.

Put aside the legality of this next comment because it is for illustration purposes. If you give all police officers a fantastic deal and they show up a few times every month, you should have a bunch of happy customers. These happy customers have an added advantage of being movers and shakers, active in your community, have lots of face time with others, and so the hope and expectation is that the police will be a big referral generator. Lose money on the front end but gain respect and help out an officer and in exchange they refer people to the clinic who pay regular fees. The problem with this clinic was that all these people with good deals were not referring.

In fact, the doctor was spending a lot of time each week on these types of visits and if you crunch the numbers, the doctor was technically losing money each time they came in. Once I caught on, I raised the price and 90% of them left because they didn't value the treatment they were receiving. In hindsight, I could have done a few things differently so more would have stuck around. I could have spent more time asking them questions about why they get treatment, what's the benefit to their health and their life, and what they would do if they didn't have it. Were they in active pain each week, or strictly maintaining their spinal and nerve health to boast their health potential? Once you gather all the facts, maybe there was a trend and then I could have addressed issues head on.

Ultimately, it would mean charging the higher price regardless of whether it was a slow or overnight transition. A popular saying, Like attracts Like, also stands true in referrals. People getting deals refer people who want deals and that doesn't really help your situation. People who have shoulder pain tend to hang out and refer other friends with shoulder pain.

At the time, I talked to people about what to do, so I'm going to assume that the approach I used and the letter we crafted to inform them of the policy changes was appropriate. The good news is that those 10% that saw the value in my chiropractic services staid and paid and I still saw them for periodic adjustments six years later.

Those first couple years, especially those first six months, were rough. One month I could pay the bills, the next month I was loading up the credit cards, one month I finally had enough profit to pay my salary, but I better be cheap because I was low last month and could dip again next month. Opening a business has lots of highs and lows and it takes time to build a solid base to have consistency. Some people are amazing; as soon as the doors are open, they just make gold out of everything they touch, but in my experience, and with most of my colleagues, that was the exception, not the norm. Again, I found myself having to scrape by and figure out how to live life on a tight budget. It took a while to go from cheap to frugal.

Cheap vs. Frugal

Cheap is looking for the lowest price regardless of quality. A cheap person might go out with friends and purposely not bring enough money to cover a tip. That was not me, just to clarify. Seriously though, being cheap might mean you go without material possessions for the sake of not spending money. You may buy an inferior product that breaks way too soon and needs to be replaced again. So much for being cheap: you spend money on junk for round one and you either replace it with junk or cough up the money for the more expensive, better quality one. If you had just bought the better quality product for an extra 20%, you would be better off. I'm not saying buy the highest price version, but one in the midrange is a good compromise. I think there comes a point where the price doesn't outweigh the benefits, and often it's because it has some fancy brand name attached to it.

Frugal is looking for that quality product, but saving money by searching for a deal. I like to walk 10,000+ steps a day and that means I want a good pair of shoes so my feet and knees won't hurt. Plus, I need them to last for more than three months. A frugal person will still buy a top rated shoe but instead of it being the current model, he/she will do a search online and find last year's top product. Why not get an awesome shoe for a huge discounted rate? You think people really A) care what your wearing that much or B) have any clue what year your shoes came out? The answer is no, so why not pick up the top rated running shoe from the previous year for 65% off the current model's price.

Frugal people go to restaurants and pay for tax and tip like a good customer, but save money by skipping a fancy drink and appetizer. Instead of buying one drink at a bar, they gather at a friend's house to watch the big game and buy a whole six pack for a buck more. Maybe they cook their own chicken wings and create three of their own sauces they found recipes for online.

After six months, the frugal person might then take all their smart spending choices savings and go on a vacation. The cheap person stays at home complaining that spending money on a vacation is such a waste.

I saw a video that compared three stainless steel mugs. One was around $50, the other $25, and the winner was a $9 identical rip-off of the most expensive model. The main difference was the ice lasted longer on the least costly model but the trade-off is that for those people who care about brands would scoff at you and your family of four will each have one. I guess the joke is on them.

My point is simple. Some people who have your same salary will spend more money on brands, eat out several times a week, buy multiple drinks at a bar, buy the newest car every two years, and find themselves in a financial hole. They probably are taking the same vacations as you are too but the credit card bill just keeps inflating, whereas your vacation is paid for in cash. The frugal budget conscious person will not over spend their salary and could have the same fancy brands because of how they shopped for them and enjoy that same vacation. Being frugal doesn't mean outlandish sacrifice, it just means shopping smarter.

These days, I spend similar amounts of my salary compared to my peers, but the main question is, are you spending your time and money on what you find most important? I value travel and I plan my life so I can do more of that. If you are into car restoration, you might divert your savings so you can afford the new turbo charger and upgraded suspension for your next car show in Biloxi. For a long while, I pinched pennies because I had to. When I could loosen the grip and be purposely frugal, it was a process to let go and learn how.

The Value of Relationships and Money

Relationships with significant others can be harmed not only by over spending but also being overly stingy. This isn't a relationship advice book, but I will throw in this nugget for you. Don't nitpick everything your spouse buys; Why did you get coffee? You spent $20 on a pair of shoes? Did you need another box of fishing lures? Instead, save yourselves a lot of fights and come up with an allowance based on your budget that each of you can spend each month on whatever you want, no questions asked. For example: each of you has $100 to spend on whatever suites you. If he spends it all on a new remote control (which you think is stupid) and she spends it on her nails and a paint and drink wine party (which you think is outrageous), you both can do it and the other can't say anything. It's just an easy way to have some autonomy without having to justify every purchase to someone. As that old joke says, "But baby I saved 50%!" "But baby you still spent $60."

If you are sticking to a tight budget because your debt is out of control or for whatever reason really, then you will recognize that fights occur because of these small purchases. We don't tend to criticize our own splurges, do we? You buying another pair of yoga pants might sound like a good reason to get angry but she might be just as angry with your new Bluetooth speaker or the overpriced protein shakes from the gym. Oh yes, we don't want to look in the mirror and see our own purchases as frivolous.

If I gave you $100 at the end of the month, what would you do with it? Would you pay down debt, replace the microwave, save it for a vacation, or maybe put it in an IRA? Five dollars a day per person is $300 at the end of the month. Wouldn't it be better to set an allowance as part of the budget, rather than fight about purchases and spend over $10 a day on average? I hope you are following my logic. If you set an allowance of $200 in the budget, then you will not mindlessly spend over that amount in a month. It's very easy to spend a little here and a little there and the average daily expenses were $300 or more by the end of the month. The budget puts restraints on what you can spend, so you just gave yourself $100 at the end of the month to do what you want with.

My advice again is to have an agreed upon amount that each of you can spend per month without having to be held accountable to each other. He can spend $100 on protein shakes at the gym and you can think that's silly because he isn't using the milk and protein powder in the fridge for a fraction of the cost. You don't say anything, don't judge, and don't harbor resentment. The caveat is that he has to realize that if by the 20th of the month he spent all of the allowance, he can't spend anymore for 11 days. After a couple of months of running out of the allowance early on in the month, that person begins to make more frugal decisions. It sure can be frustrating when your spouse picks up a little something special on the 29th and you are stuck with nothing. Responsibility is learned the hard way for some people so start changing some spending habits today.

One more nugget: each family should come up with a dollar amount they feel is necessary to get others' approval prior to purchasing. Every budget is different but let's agree that anything over $100 for a single item might cause your significant other to say a few choice words. Therefore, the significant other needs to be consulted for anything over $100 and both must agree to buy it. For instance, the house needs a new fancy mop and it costs $50. You buy it and there's no real issue. The mop is something the household needs for sanitary reasons and doesn't come from anyone's allowance. Remember, time is one of our most valuable assets and a good mop system might save you a lot of time cleaning. We each get 24 hours a day to spend, so spend it wisely (and yes sleeping 6-8 hours is valuable).

Let's say you find a mop for $125. If your family set a partner approval for any purchase over $100, then you would need to talk to your spouse about it. Every family has to determine what is right for them. These pre-approval purchases will really help stop impulse buys and will make you discuss the pros and cons of each item. Do we really need this product or can it wait? Can we find a slightly less feature rich version at a better price?

Another perk is that you might just uncover the source to a lot of the money fights you've had in the past. The wife might finally recognize that she gets frustrated and resentful when her husband comes home with another electronic gadget around the $100 mark. By having a pre-approved limit, those types of purchases could be vetoed and make for a healthier marriage and bank account. Who wouldn't like to fight less and build new loving cooperative memories with their significant other?

Over the years, I've learned hard lessons on my path to frugalness. Some involved failed relationships, poor decisions in marketing that took a long time to recover from, poor choices in products, and repurchases for better quality. I can honestly say it's the tough situations in life that cause us to grow. When things are going great most people don't stop and think about how they can grow stronger financially, socially, spiritually, showing love, etc. We just coast along. No one wants to redo those low points, so learn the lessons the first time round and don't repeat them. Hire a coach or get a mentor and avoid the most common mistakes people make. When you hit a hurdle (because no matter how successful you are, you will always have struggles), ask for their advice and overcome it quicker and with wisdom. Some mistakes can cost you your career, your family, or take years to pay back, so try to seek wise counsel and avoid being unethical.

These past few pages paint a picture of struggles, growth, and practical applications. I share this background so you can better understand that even though I don't have an economics degree (you should always seek professional help when making big financial decisions), I think my experience can alter your course.

Living a life on a budget for the past 15 years gives me credibility. During my years of clinic ownership in Colorado, every Thursday morning I sat down on Quickbooks® and input all my expenses, because I wanted to track where the money was going. If I was over budget, I could see it immediately and figure out why: did the X-ray processor go out, were vitamins got reordered, or was it a pretty standard month... because I track it, I can know. If money was leaving my bank then I wrote it down and could graph it to look for inconsistencies and trends.

Overspending typically occurs thanks to emergencies, but hopefully with this book's help, you can set up an emergency fund so you don't have to sacrifice so much when they come up. I enjoyed those Thursday mornings and comparing one month to the last month and the same time period of the previous year. In business, I always checked to see if this April was the same, better, or worse than last year's April. My goal was to grow. On the personal side, I was also looking to see if my lifestyle increased over the past year, and if so, by what percentage. Maybe I could have been an accountant if I didn't love chiropractic so much.

You can also budget for expenses you know only happen once per year. For example, getting your fire extinguishers checked yearly, your high school teenager needs an outfit for prom, best friend gets married in the summer etc. When you know that extra $100 is coming up, you can plan accordingly months prior. Don't forget gifts and weddings will happen every year, so just add that as an item in your budget to save for.

How did I overspend so much? Now what?

STEP 1: Gathering the Information

If tracking all these expenses by hand sounds overwhelming, boring, and you would rather give up now than even try...then hang on a second. Not everyone wants to be the next Quickbooks or PeachTree expert (nor pay for it) so I get it. There are other options out there that can import all your bank account and credit card statements automatically and some do it for free. All you do is follow their steps to link your accounts and all your purchases and deposits get automatically put into their program. Research several sites because most are only allowed to read your statements. The good ones, in my opinion, are not allowed to actually touch your money via transfers.

Sometimes you have to go through and change an expense (bill) category or add one when they can't figure out what the purchase was for, but that's just a minor detail. For instance, if you went to a place called Rad Rats, the program might enter it as a pet store or as unclassified. You just have to change it to Auto Repair because this auto mechanic named their business Rad Rats.

Most of these programs allow you to type in a budget per category (food, car, insurance, etc.) and track with numbers, bars, and graphs (for visual people), and how you are doing in each category. You can see in an instant that you are over budget in the entertainment category but you still have $50 left in charitable donations. Mint.com is the website I use for this process and it is owned by Quickbooks (which I also use and trust). There are other options and I encourage you to find one that you trust and will actually use. Most of these websites even have phone apps. A quick internet search using phrases like:

Mint vs. ___ or Mint vs. free budget trackers should give you a good start to reading up on the various options.

Take a deep breath. Breathe in for four seconds; out for four seconds; repeat four times. Now that your heart rate is reduced, your muscles are relaxed, and freshly oxygenated blood has entered your brain, let's jump into the budget making process. I realize a budget can sound stuffy and overly restrictive, but if your finances are in shambles, maybe it's time to get serious.

Another aspect of hesitance is past mistakes. When we are brave enough to put all of our bills on paper, suddenly the truth is staring at us and most of us don't like confrontation. No more running. It is all right there—all the victories and all the embarrassment. Don't worry, the past is done. We can't change the past but we can change the now.

Unfortunately, our past spending faux pas can stay with us for years. Have you ever bought a boat? Did you realize you would also incur all the accessory payments too: docking fees, fishing license, insurance, winterizing, maintenance, plus any damages and sports equipment? A few years go by and that boat stays docked all but twice a year. Finally you sell it at a loss just to stop bleeding money season after season. At this point, you are out thousands of dollars on a purchase that stopped giving you pleasure years ago. To make matters worse, it's not uncommon for other bills to have piled up from eating out and that new truck payment you acquired to haul that boat you no longer want.

Some reading this may not relate to such a big purchase. Here's a classic freshman in college mistake that you might relate to better because this could be your story or you know "that person." Just a normal Wednesday afternoon walking to the student union for a light lunch when suddenly a noisy crowd of people catches your attention. You see over 20 people waiting in line with clipboards, and smiles and pens filling out some kind of application. It just so happens that the banner hanging over the front of the line is showcasing the rival football game on Saturday and you can get a free t-shirt and koozie. That's stupid, you say, I'm hungry, but next thing you know XYZ credit card company has your name, address, and a signature. One week later, you get that credit card with your school mascot emblazoned on the front with a spending limit of $2,500. It goes in your billfold, not because you plan on using it, but for showing your friends and 'just in case' an emergency happens. A few months later, the late night clubbing, big sale on shoes, eating out, and the latest video game finally catches up with you. A variation of the following takes place. The grocery cart is full of frozen pizzas, bananas, milk, bread, PB&J fixings, and the cashier says that'll be $45.87, please. Your scratched up mascot card gets swiped and declined. The bagged groceries are left at the counter, you leave humiliated, and confirm via a phone call that Yes, indeed the card is working properly, but you have maxed out the $2,500 limit. Two questions are tossed around your head. How did this emergency only credit card get maxed out? How in the crap am I going to pay for this?

Are you a bad person, a failure because of these two scenarios? No, definitely not. I've heard this quoted many times on podcasts. There are no successes or failures in life, only results based on choices made. Sometimes our choices lead to poor results and sometimes they lead to amazing, profitable results. Were you mindlessly spending and irresponsible with money? YES. Hopefully, you learned a lesson through that experience. By the way, how did you pay it back? Did your family bail you out or did you get a job making minimum wage? I hope you picked a job and realized that, at 23% interest, your better put all the money you can to paying this card off, otherwise you'll still owe on it 10 years later.

The best option is not to make that mistake to begin with and definitely not do it again. Maybe after reading this book, you can help your family, children, and friends to avoid similar mistakes. Financial literacy is one of the most important lessons you can learn and it's not taught in school. Our kids can be saved a lot of drama in adulthood if we teach them sound financial principles early in life. We all know people who spend all their money regardless of income level. When you make $30,000 a year, you might buy used vehicles, coupon shop, furnish a 1000 sq. ft. house, go to the movies, and only have a few pennies to rub together at the end of the month. Someone who makes $300,000 can still be broke because they upgraded to brand furniture, a 3,500 sq. ft. house, luxury car and clothes, and eat at fancy restaurants several times a week.

Many people who start earning more money end up increasing their cost of living. One day, you are eating fast food ($7), the next day it's a mom and pop place ($10), then it's a big box restaurant chain ($15), and finally it becomes the more expensive places ($20-50). It all boils down to one principle: we are just one paycheck away from ruin. The only sum that matters is what you save at the end of the month, not what you made. Imagine making $80,000 but only living on half of it. That's a great amount of savings, plus less headaches and stress each month.

The phrase, "one paycheck away from ruin" has a simple meaning. Regardless of income, if you spend 99% of it by the end of the month, it will only take 1-2 months to go broke if you lost your job. This means, if you lost your job, then that next paycheck will be missing and you can't pay the bills because you only saved 1% of your salary each month. Even having three months of expenses in your bank account runs out quickly if you can't find a job and everything you own is locked into a fixed payment for the next couple of years.

When you subtract all your mandatory monthly payments, some really only have 15% or less of their income for food, electricity, and entertainment. I would venture to say many don't even have half a month of savings. Which again means, if you owe $1,500 to the bank each month and you only have $300 to your name, what are you going to do to meet that deficit? If you don't pay and get behind even further, then you get the privilege of owing even more money due to late fees and penalties. Next thing you know you are getting Final Notice letters, repossessions, and eventually may have to file bankruptcy (which ruins you for seven years).

It's much harder to scale back your spending and lifestyle after being accustomed to a way of life for such a long time but hopefully you can see the virtue of living with a fixed budget and ample savings each month. Make a pledge to go through the process outlined in this section and break the cycle. The hole you dug yourself might take years to get out of, but you can do it, one back-breaking shovelful at a time. Luckily, you now know a chiropractor! You may never know just how capable you are to fix the situation if you don't do the work to find out. Go through the process, learn something about yourself, but please take action.

Phase 2 of Step 1: Write it down

Now is the time to start recording your expenses/ bills. If you don't record them, you can't track and measure them so you can't make appropriate modifications on your spending habits. As previously mentioned, an automatic website makes it really easy to track. It already has categories and your bank and credit card statements are automatically put into the budget tracking website in the appropriate category. After a month, you can click a button and see a graph on how much you are actually spending versus what you think you're spending in all the different categories so you can see your Spent vs. What's Left in each category.

Cash is the only way to cheat, so don't let that happen. An ice cream cone through the drive thru that costs $1.07 needs to be tracked. That's over $30 at the end of the month. If your situation is that bad, think of that $30 as one less minimum payment on a credit card. In a year, that is $360 of undocumented expenses and is arguably 1-6 months of payments you could have erased if you paid that into your debt. You can use cash; all I am asking is that you record it. Unfortunately, you will have to log in to the account and do it yourself.

Gather your paychecks for the last three months

This portion is all dependent on how you get paid. If you get paid once a month and it's the same day every month, then just look at that deposit and record it on a sheet of paper as Income. Use a heading like Main Job or Name of Company I work for. If you get paid the same amount twice a month, again add up the amount and write it down. Write down how much you were paid from your main job over the past three months.

Those who work commission, tips, or work hourly plus overtime pay should do the following. Look at your pay stubs, cash tips, bank deposits...pretty much be as honest and thorough as possible in adding up your income. Go back for three months and add them all up. Once you have the big total, divide by three. Now you have an average amount you earned per month. Why do an average? Because I know one week you may get paid a ton, and the next you can barely get by. The average gives you a general idea of what you will and should make each month so you can create a budget later in the book.

If you have several jobs, keep each income recording separate. Main job, Second job, Lawn Mowing on Saturday etc. should all have their own line under the income heading. This exercise might surprise you as to which job you make the most money at versus the time spent. This will come in handy later on. It might look something like this.

INCOME

Main Job/ Teacher	$3,000
Second Job/ Mowing Grass	$220
Third Job/ Babysitting	$80
Fourth Job/ Tutoring	$700
TOTAL	$4,000

Write down your expenses

Be diligent when combing through your credit card statements, bank statements, checks, cash receipts, and think about what you didn't keep a receipt for. The computer programs should be able to go back a month or two if you search the site and figure out how. Whatever the max timeframe your bank allows you to see without having to download an official PDF is what the programs will upload automatically. My bank does 90 days so technically mint.com could pull three months of past transactions for me to immediately see trends.

Our discussion in this book will be for those who use pen and paper. I encourage you to go old school even if you use a program because there is a proven level of learning when you write things down, not just looking on a screen. Plus, as I will discuss later, you may need to break down some of your purchases, like at Costco, into more detailed categories and it will be easier to do on paper.

Reality check: Do the best you can to go back at least the past 30 days. Some people have such horrible records that going back two or three months will be nearly impossible. Most people throw away receipts, especially cash purchases, so the past months will probably be way off. If you fall into this category, then just do the present month from whatever day it is now. Continue to track for the current month and the next two months. Better late than never... but not too late.

Get a few sheets of paper and start listing categories. Feel free to just list the categories I provide in a few pages. Write each one and go down three inches and write another. Add space so you have room to record the numbers.

No lumping together, Point 1

Try not to lump all auto expenses under the heading AUTO EXPENSE. Break it down into Auto, indent one inch: gasoline, oil changes, car wash, and repairs. For INSURANCE, try breaking it down into: auto insurance, boat insurance, house insurance, and life insurance. Make sense?

When you have a big total for AUTO of $500 one month, you won't really know where the money went exactly. Maybe you had to buy a tire and an oil change. An oil change is only once every few months so you can take that $30 and spread it out over four months. Now the Auto category will have a more realistic amount per month without the shock when you need your oil changed or new tires. When you average out the total Auto Expense for the year, it will balance out, even though you are under budget every three months and are over budget one month in this category. By the end of the year, it will be accurate...you only wanted to spend $120 on oil changes for the year and you did (even though the amount actually spent was $0 most months). The point is that you aren't judging what you will spend based on how much money is in your bank account, but rather you only spend what your budget tells you to. Our budgets will obviously not allow us to spend more money than we earn.

Point 2

The second important point when recording your expenses (bills) is to break up the total bill into smaller categories when shopping at mega stores like Target®, Costco®, and Walmart® with groceries, auto, sports, hygiene products, washing machines, jewelry, entertainment and more. You can buy stuff in each of these categories in one visit. So just lumping the entire bill under one category isn't accurate.

You should be diligent, honest, and do a good job. It's a lot of detailed work to go through each receipt and break the bill down to appropriate categories. If all you have is a bill on your automated computer program or bank statement that says Target $247.35, that won't be very helpful. If you notice you do all your shopping at mega stores and you don't keep the receipts, then you can't break down your bills into categories for the past months. The best you can hope for is the last week or two. A grand total is better than nothing, but please, keep your receipts starting today so you can properly categorize your purchases for the next three months.

For now, if you have bad records, you can still compare the current and last months' total balances to figure out the general amount you are spending each month and where. Most people are consistent in their spending. If you are consistently over budget by $100, it will probably be somewhat the same, unless you had an emergency that put you in the hole even more than usual.

Method 1: Broken down correctly with receipts

MEGA STORE Receipt Total $245	Broken down correctly
Subcategory	
Auto	$15 (air filter)
Clothes	$30 (exercise pants)
Entertainment	$20 (2 for 1 movie)
Grocery	$180 (why you actually went)

Method 2: Guessing the amount you spent based on a percentage because you only have grand totals

MEGA STORE Receipt $245	As a guessing percent, which is not as accurate
Subcategory	
Auto	5% = 12
Clothes	5% = 12
Entertainment	15% = 37
Grocery	75% = 184

Method 2 is for those who have poor receipts to look back on, so you can think about what you typically buy at a mega store. Maybe 70% is food and 30% is paper towels and bug spray. If you have a good handle on your typical shopping trip, you can split that bill into smaller categories even without a detailed receipt.

New Month- Current Day to Day Bills.

You have to keep detailed receipts even after three months.

After three months, you should have a handle on what you spend and we can begin looking for ways to reduce spending. You still need to write down all your expenses and put them into the categories though. The only way to get out of debt is to stop spending more than you make and use the surplus to pay off debt. You can even do a rapid debt payoff, which I will touch on later.

For the next three months, every last dime you spend should be recorded. The dollar at the drive thru needs to be written down with accuracy just like the credit card purchase of lunch and the food bill at the neighborhood organic grocery store. Record the bills each day. At the end of the month, just add the subcategories to get a total. Then add those together for a total in each main category and circle it. Then add up circled totals from each category and write that as Grand Total. There are plenty free budget templates online with pre-populated categories. Each day, just add a few new rows and you can have a detailed, accurate expense list.

STEP 2: Compare Income vs. Expenses

It's time to compare your total income to total expenses. You might find it helpful to use an average of the three months before doing this step. Do the averages based on the subcategories and add them for your categories and the grand total.

Month 1:	charities 200,	church 100
Subcategory		
Month 2:	charities 100,	church 200
Month 3:	charities 75,	church 150

Charity 200+100+75=375 375/3= 125

$125 average of 3 months given to charity

Church 100+200+150=450 450/3=150

$150 average of 3 months given to church

150+125=275

Therefore the **category Giving** has an average of $275 per month.

Compare income to expenses when the categories and grand totals are averaged.

Food	Auto
Alcohol (general a waste of $)	Car replacement
Fast food	Fuel
Grocery	License plate
Restaurant	Maintenance
Tobacco (waste of $ & kills)	Oil change
Utilities	Parking fees
Electricity	Repairs
Heating/gas	Tires
Trash	Insurance
Water	Auto
House/ Rent	Boat etc.
Technology	Disability insurance
Cell phone	Homeowner's/Renter
Internet	Identity theft
WIFI	protection

Giving
  Charities
  Church
  Politics

Savings/ Retirement
  College fund
  401K
  Regular savings for emergency fund
  Roth IRA

Entertainment
  Concerts
  Hobby
  Movie at theater
  Movie Rental
  Music
  Painting
  Sporting Events
  TV subscriptions

Allowance
  His/hers
  Kids

Miscellaneous Fees
  ATM
  Bank fees
  Late fees credit cards

Hygiene
  Cosmetics

Life insurance
Long-term care

Medical
  Chiropractor
  Co-pays
  Insurance Premium
  Deductible
  Dental
  Eye doctor
  Not covered services

Debt
  Bank Loan for car
  Credit card A
  Credit card B
  Student loan

Sports
  Equipment
  Gym membership

Gifts
  Anniversary
  Birthdays
  Christmas
  Weddings

Vacations

Education
  Books
  Daycare
  Kid's school tuition

Cleaning supplies
Detergents
Hair cuts
Soap/shampoo
	School supplies
	
	Clothing
	  Business
	  Children
	  Jewelry
	  Personal

This part is simple. Is your income higher than your expenses? Is it less? How much difference? The amount that you are short each month is called a deficit. The extra amount is called a surplus.

Congrats, you just finished step 2. Grab another sheet of paper and answer the following questions.
What are your thoughts and emotions after doing this exercise?
If you feel sad or disappointed, write that down.
Are you frustrated, content, optimistic: write that down.
Don't stop there though. Explain why you feel that way.
Sometimes writing things down helps you move on and relieves stress.
Are you happy with the results or disappointed?
Were you surprised? Why were you surprised?
Did you learn anything?
Where can you do better?
What is the number one emotion you are experiencing now?
Are you blaming someone else for the mess of your financial life?
What is your role in the current situation?
Are you super excited about how well you are doing?
Can you give thanks to anyone for helping you in this area of life?
For those who have been on a plan before reading this book, where have you seen improvements from one month, three months or even a year ago?

Has anyone been a mentor in your life that you want to give thanks to?

I challenge you to really answer these questions. Some people are afraid to sit and explore the deeper connections and meanings in their life. Nothing scares them more than dealing with their past and their own demons. Own your successes and failures and take steps to keep moving forward. So many times we have poor relationships with money (and body image for that matter) due to our past. If you know you have some issues that changed the course of your life, I encourage you to deal with them and not let them control your life anymore. Don't be afraid to explore your childhood, the relationship with your parents, coaches growing up, and how you and your friends interacted with each other.

Psychologists are available if you need expert advice on any trauma and other issues you may be dealing with. Remember you are not alone; you are not the only one who has ever dealt with these issues. I can promise you, there is nothing you can say that they haven't already heard.

Journaling

Have you ever had so much to do the next day that you can't shut your brain off to sleep? You keep waking up all night and the next day you're grumpy and tired and underperform at your tasks. Well, one way to cure such an unpleasant situation is to write down whatever is on your mind. Have a notebook or a journal and keep it near your bed with a pen. If you find yourself stressed out and your brain is racing, write down everything that comes to mind.

Is it a "to do" list that you don't want to forget? Write it down and now you don't have to think about it. Anytime during the night or even the next day, when you notice yourself getting anxious about remembering what to do, just read it back to yourself. No more reciting the 10 things on your list, and stressing out because you forgot number 8. Refer back to the list anytime you need to.

Another aspect of journaling is the Habit of Gratitude. You can write down all the positive things that happened that day. Positive affirmations about yourself, family, and friends can be written down too. To look back six months from now and see where you have been and where you are now is an extraordinary gift. Were you struggling with depression and now you aren't? Did you have bouts of low self-esteem because of money troubles? Now when you journal, you may notice that it's a happy journal post because you aren't a slave to a credit card anymore. Sometimes you find that what seemed like a mountain before was actually just a hill half its size.

I listen to a lot of podcasts where extremely successful people are interviewed. Journaling, usually just five minutes a day (usually when they wake up and sometimes five minutes before bed), is something they all do. They swear it's one of the best habits they have. It clears their head and focuses them on what is important for today (meetings, being creative, making time to see the kids play sports) and reflect back on what was actually most important in their life (how they treated people, did family time enrich their lives, did they land that big job, how were they thankful today and did they show gratitude to others).

Take the time to evaluate your emotions and write down positives and negatives of your day. You can even write down short-term goals (next week or month), mid-term goals (1-2 years from now) and long-term goals (5+years from now). It's amazing how writing down goals and looking at them every day/week is a huge step in actually achieving them. When you read your goals often, they become a part of you and you find ways to take steps towards those goals. We often aren't even aware what we want in life and even if the perfect opportunity arose, we wouldn't notice it. Great experiences can be lost because of lack of planning.

STEP 3: Evaluate Overspending and Reduce It

This is the fun step. You can get creative in many ways to reduce spending. I will give you a handful of examples and more importantly, <u>concepts</u> to help you make choices on saving money. If you need more inspiration, check the internet because there are so many blogs available on how to coupon shop, budget, how to save money on everyday purchases, negotiating fees, low cost to zero cost dates, etc.

What are the top three areas you spend the most on? Can you reduce them?

Eating out, entertainment, clothes shopping, and insurance might be some easy areas to look at. Another bigger area to consider is downgrading your car and house to really save big chunks of money. Be patient and I'll cover those two as well.

I will cover the following areas because it seems most people over =spend in them: eating out, insurance, dates, cars, electronics, clothes, and a couple of wonderful tangents.

As a general rule of thumb, <u>each category of expenses should only be spent at a maximum percentage of your income</u>. You don't want your house to cost 60% of your income and the car taking up another 30%. How do you live on 10%?

Here is a typical breakdown:

Income Percentage For Each Expense Category	
car expenses	10-15%
charity	4-10%
clothing	4%
entertainment	5%
food	14%
house	24-34%
medical	6-9%
savings	5-10%
personal debt	12%
utilities	8%

Dates

Have you ever heard of the dating term "one and done?" Research tells us that we size people up on nonverbal cues within the first three seconds we meet someone. When you shake someone's hand for the first time, have you ever felt like this person was a sleaze ball and just didn't trust him/her. If so, and I know you have, then you experienced that initial judgment of someone. In fact, even if you met someone who you immediately admired and then they hurt your trust, you will still find them somewhat trustworthy compared to a negative first impression of someone who does amazing things for you, yet it's still difficult to like them because of that first impression.

First impressions can change but it takes time to change your mind on a more permanent basis. Anyway, if you are single and going on a date, you want your first impression to be stellar.

Then you can talk and get to know each other.

In an effort to meet new people outside of my friend circle, I did online dating. I wanted it to be successful so I read a few posts online about it. Then I talked to people who have tried it (mostly women to find out the do's and don'ts) and some men (find out what to look out for), and I was given some good advice.

You can usually tell if a date is going to go well or not within the first 10 minutes. This means you don't want to be stuck in some long date if you are already ready to go. They also said maybe don't take the girl out to a restaurant because you might be stuck for an hour with someone you don't find interesting and then have to pay for it. Paying for meals out twice a week every week turns into a lot of money at the end of the month. It's also a lot of wasted money if you are only doing one date. Hence the term, one and done.

Some people don't even date because they say they can't afford to. If you think you need to spend $40 every time you go out, of course you can't afford that. Here are some tricks you can use as a single person and even as an adult to save money. Take the other person out for coffee. It's only $3 instead of $15. Plus, the added bonus is that in 30 minutes you can politely excuse yourself and move on with your day if neither of you is feeling the vibe. Another option is to go on a lunch date because you will have to go to work in an hour and you can get lunch time specials. Maybe go to a park and a walk. The idea of dating your spouse or someone new is all about communicating, what better way than at a park? Teach the other person a new sport or exercise. The bonding that takes place is incredible.

Movie Theater

Going to a movie theater gets expensive. You can't talk, the tickets are high priced, and don't even get me started on concession stand food. If you want to see the latest movie with the big sound system, then catch a matinee for the lower price. It's a pretty cool feeling walking out of a movie and being blinded by sunlight. I feel like I have a brand new day, two days in one. Also, shop around to find a theater that is cheaper. There aren't many Dollar Theater's left, but when I was in Colorado I found one that was half the normal price and still had new releases. Other discount places have an older movie selection. Whatever you do, do not buy concession food. $7 is way too much for popcorn and $5 for a soda is a rip off. Are you really that hungry and thirsty? Do you really think these indulgences are good for your waist line either? Eat before you go. I can hear you whine, "But I like the snacks and that's part of the whole movie-going experience." Being financially smart takes sacrifices, and for some of you, that sacrifice is saving $20 at the theater and being snack free. Maybe just skip the theater all together and rent a movie.

Cable and Wi-Fi

Cut the cable bill and just pay for Wi-Fi. Find out what the latest streaming movie site requires for no buffering and only subscribe to that much Wi-Fi speed. Hulu®, Fox®, ABC®, NBC®, Netflix® etc. all stream their TV shows online. Just wait a few days after it airs and you can watch it, many times for free. After the initial delay, you can stay caught up each week and still discuss the show around the water cooler. These days, you can attach cables from your computer to your TV or maybe you have a smart TV with built-in Wi-Fi. Now you can't complain about watching TV on your computer and you are still utilizing your 60 inch TV. A Hulu and Netflix subscription is still cheaper than cable. There are also products from Google®, Apple®, Amazon® and Roku® to watch even more affordable TV. If you have to watch more sports than available, talk to a friend and have a party. Seriously, you get 2-3 free games on Saturday and Sunday and another free one at least once in the weekday. Seems like enough time spent on a recliner to me.

Gym Membership

Is it time to evaluate your gym membership? The biggest waste of money is having a gym membership and not using it. As a health goal, you need to be in there four times a week. As I said, start slow; I don't care if you are in there for only 20 minutes a day for the first month. The important thing is that you are building a routine and prepping your body.

Now some of us have a card at the best gym in town. Why? Even if you are using it, can you get out of the contract and go somewhere less expensive? I understand a lot of places have you sign a year contract, so leaving now may not make much sense. Nobody wants to waste $250 on an early termination fee.

You would have to save at least 1.5x the termination fee broken down into 12 months for it to be worth it. Plus, you have to consider the enrollment fee at the new place. If the fee is $250 then 250*1.5=375: 375/12= 31.25: the new enrollment fee is $99: 99/12=8.25; you would have to save 31.25+8.25= $39.50 per month in your new gym's monthly membership rate for it to be worth it. Good luck!

Just go to the gym you are already paying for and get the most out of your buck. Every time you walk in the doors, you are lowering the average cost per visit. I remember during chiropractic school, I bought a two-year plan up front because my friends were going too. Well, I think each workout I did was nearly $400 because I didn't go. That was a waste of money. Can you sacrifice the racquet ball court and pool and go to a gym with a fewer amenities? Sure you can.

If you are looking for a gym in the first place, find one that has the cardio equipment you like (maybe elliptical machines) and has quality, safe weight lifting machines. Find one that is convenient to either work or home. You won't use it if it takes all day to get there and back. Check online and the newspaper for free or heavily discounted enrollment and any specials. Some gyms let you go free or cheaply for one week to test it out. Pick the best gym that you will actually use. Final tip, ask what the family rates are. They almost always have a good deal for a family.

Electronics

Electronics are typically a guy's worst enemy. The new shiny object comes out and suddenly you have 20 reasons why you need the upgraded version. Worse yet, you now must have this new invention you never even knew existed until today.

Really investigate your cell phone bill. How much data are you really using? Can you reduce it? Are you streaming music and videos without Wi-Fi? STOP IT! The phone companies make a killing on your data plans so if you can just stream on Wi-Fi think about how much money you can save as an individual and as a family. Get on a family plan. Some places only add $10 to your bill, which is way better than a starting rate of $50+ individually. Remember that the government has mandated that you can keep your number.

Don't upgrade your phone too often. The new model came out last week, so what? How different is it? Regardless, your phone works. Keep the phone for at least two years. Even if you get a good deal on the phone by signing a contract, you will still pay $200, which is still $17 a month. If you were to write a $17 check every month to a company, I have a strong hunch that we would all think twice about purchasing the most high tech phone out there every year.

With that said, if you are in the market for a new phone and the 7 just came out, go check out the 6 because the price will be less and will have almost the same features. I highly recommend buying a really good protective case for your phone and don't be afraid to spend $40-75. This is a cheap insurance policy for your $700 phone. We all drop our phones, so don't risk breaking it because you put in a plastic glitter case. With a proper case like Otterbox® or Life Proof®, you can drop it without it breaking. That saves you $100 fixing the screen, even more if the phone's internals break, and it saves the aggravation if you choose not to fix it and live with a broken screen.

A tech friend of mine was walking around with no case and I asked him, "Are you crazy?" He had a great answer, but he still decided to buy a case a few months later. Here is the advice: He became aware of what he was doing when he did drop his phone. Then he quit doing it. He always had a stack of stuff in his hands while going to his car. On the way to the car, he would place the phone on top of the stack. When he leaned over to get into the car, the phone would slide across the papers and hit the ground. Solution: He put the phone in his pocket until he got in the car, so he no longer dropped it. Figure out where/ how you are clumsy and remedy the situation.

I only mentioned phones but this can apply to just about any gadget. Do you really need a heart rate monitor or an electronic step counter? No, you probably don't and you can save $150 while you are at it. In fact, I would argue you don't need one at all since our phones, which are in your pocket, usually have a step counter built in.

Insurance

The bane of my existence is insurance. Not only do I have car and house, but malpractice, business and disability. These three extra expenses take a big chunk out of my income. You may know the feeling if you have an RV, ATV, and a boat.

My advice for you is mostly about making phone calls and getting quotes, but let's explore insurance. First, contact your agent and ask for all the details of your auto insurance: comprehensive, collision, deductible, insured motorist, glass, roadside assistance, MedPay and whatever else has a dollar figure to it. Second, ask the agent where you can save money without compromising if you got into an accident.

One of the quickest ways to reduce your premium is to raise that deductible to a rate you can afford to spend if you got in an accident. Maybe you are a safe driver and you are ok with spending $1,000 instead of $500 if you get in an accident. Typically, there are big savings between those two numbers. The jump to $1,500 isn't usually as much of a saving from $1,000 over the course of a year and then you're still another $500 out of pocket. In my opinion, I would want to save $500 on the deductible per year along with the decrease in premium from the $1,000 amount. Make your own decision on that one.

Playing around with the comprehensive (comp) and collision amounts will also save you money. Just remember that the higher you put in, the more risk you take even if you are saving money. **Be careful not to be cheap and sacrifice the whole point of insurance.** Third, make sure you have all your insurable items with one company. Discounts for car and house are a standard so make sure you check.

Do you have a kid in school who makes good grades, do you drive very low miles per year, do you own more cars than you can drive at one time, how old are you, and have you taken a defensive driving course? If you answered yes to any of these questions, then you could qualify for a discount.

When you know all the particulars about your current insurance carrier, it's time to make some phone calls. Call at least three other companies and ask for a quote based on the coverage you are actually paying for right now. Some companies will say 'oh yea we can save you $75 a month' but you don't read the fine print and you realize that they removed uninsured motorist and MedPay or did some other sneaky thing and now you have worse coverage. Again, don't be too cheap and find out you have a $2,000 deductible that you can't afford to spend on fixing your crashed car when what you really wanted was a $1,000 deductible.

Approach your house insurance with the same type of questions. There are not as many variables but deductible is a big one. Make sure that if your house was destroyed by a natural disaster, you are paying enough insurance to actually cover the cost to rebuild. If you have fancy jewelry, art work, or other high end items, be sure to ask about special add-on policies in case they get destroyed too. How upsetting would it be if your $10,000 ring was stolen while you slept only to find out your basic home policy only covers $5,000 total.

While listening to a podcast I heard of a company that tailors plans to those people who can afford $100,000 pieces of artwork in their million plus 5,000 sq. ft. home. This company's office is decorated with paintings and statues that cost between

$50,000-300,000. How do they manage such an exorbitant value of collectible items? Every piece of art is valued at Zero Dollars because they are all damaged and can't be sold. In the lobby is a huge glass sculpture with a visible crack in the middle. This $100,000 specially commissioned sculpture is now just a gigantic paperweight and if they didn't have it properly insured, the owner is just hosed. The company puts these damaged goods in the office so everyone remembers why they go to work each day and how what they do matters to the customer, even if their service is a premium price. All purchases have unintended costs, some are time based and some cost money.

This reminds me of a true story I heard while living in China. Some of the local businesses decided to compete only on price. You can compete on other areas as well: offering more services, better customer support, and extra special touches that command full price and even a premium price. Well, several stores started selling a new widget. This widget costs the customer $200 and the store buys it for $100. A few months go by, and one store decides to get more of the pie on widgets and cuts the price to $180. The other stores notice a drop in sales and they drop to $170 then $150. Next thing you know, all the stores sell the widget for $120 and nobody is making enough profit to want to supply that widget anymore. If you have some kind of business, consider this quick story on how you set your fees and how to value yourself to your customer versus the competition. Try and compete on something besides price.

One last gold nugget for you. You need medical coverage on your vehicle. I would recommend $5,000 of coverage. Typically, the cost is super cheap versus what you will actually receive. Some states call it MedPay. As a chiropractor and someone who has used it in the past, it is a vital component for your health after an accident. MedPay covers the medical bills after a car accident up to the amount you paid for in coverage. MRI's, Chiropractic, Physical Therapy, Massage (sometimes), and General Doctor visits can all be covered for the amount that you paid for.

It usually doesn't matter if you are at fault or not, you still get to use the money on your health. Why is this important? If the person who hits you is uninsured, your insurance will pay for your repairs. If you choose not to buy it, then you are responsible for covering your repairs. Imagine you just got hit from behind and the person was going 40 mph with no brakes pressed. Just WHAM, you are hit and your head hits the airbag and your chest is bruised from the seatbelt. The ambulance comes and off you go for an MRI of your brain. They say everything is normal, but over the next few days, your neck gets sore. A couple weeks later, you start getting headaches, and you never had headaches in your life. You were smart and didn't sign any paperwork from the insurance company that says you were ok because you heard from a friend or read this book and knew that sometimes symptoms from a car accident don't show up for a few weeks.

Side note: wait a while (maybe 4-6 weeks) if you don't immediately have symptoms from a car accident before you sign anything that says your health is fine from the accident. The last thing you want to do is sign a paper during that second week and then develop symptoms the third and you just didn't realize they came from a car accident. I see that too often, you have been warned.

Since you have headaches, you decide to go to your local friendly chiropractor to see if they can help. You go for a while and get 75% better but you plateau. The chiropractor says, "I think you need some more advanced rehab exercises because the ones I have given you aren't enough for your case." Off you go to the best physical therapist around. Three months later, you feel you are the best you are going to get and you tell all the doctors and the insurance company that you are finished with your medical treatment. Several options can happen now.

If it's your fault, you may be liable for all those bills. If it's the other person's fault and they have insurance, then you have to wait and hope their company will pay all your bills. That wait time can be as little as six months, but is usually 12-18 months. Hopefully you don't have to go to court either. The doctors can always ask you to pay upfront for treatment and have you wait for the case to settle and get reimbursed. MedPay comes to the rescue.

With MedPay, the amount you paid for is practically immediately paid to the doctor after treatment is given (usually 30 days). There is a tiered pay out, so if you had one MRI at the hospital along with an ambulance ride, then that $3,000 of bills will be paid for first. The next $2,000 will be paid to the other doctors who you saw for care. $2,000 can be spent easily: 10 visits to a chiropractor and 10 visits to a physical therapist will exhaust it. For some people, that will be enough to get the pain under control. If you were lucky and didn't need the MRI and ambulance, then you will benefit from having more visits with the chiropractor to return you to pre-accident health. You can generally rest assured that the bills will be paid very quickly regardless of whether the case goes to court or if the other was uninsured or if it was your fault. Otherwise, you may find yourself responsible for care or stressing about who will pay one year from now. Again, the quick stress free payments are only for the dollar amount you pay for (whether that's $1,000 or $10,000 of coverage).

When I was in my own accident (I got side swiped in the rain from a texting driver), I had neck and low back pain. I went to a chiropractor and a physical therapist because I know the research and didn't want long-term trouble, which is common. We all felt I was in a stable place and we ended care. I know if I exercise with poor positioning on certain positions, my C7-T1 area on the right will hurt. After an adjustment, the discomfort goes away. In fact, during my time in China, I got an MRI and found out I have a small bulge at C5. We took X-rays after the accident but an MRI wasn't warranted. I wish I knew that before I settled on the insurance payout; it would have been more. I used my MedPay and had no issues getting everyone paid.

Compare that to a guy whose case went to court two years later. He had a huge bill with me and with some other doctors. He ended up needing injections and a few other things. Anyway, they went to court, the insurance company lawyers were quite good, and the injured guy lost. Now he owed me a few thousand dollars for treatment rendered. We negotiated a discounted rate but unfortunately, he never paid and I had to send him to collections. MedPay would have covered his bills with me and his situation may have turned out better; no court, no collection agency calling, and no hit to his credit score.

Clothes

Stop paying full price for clothes. Better yet, can you just stop buying new items? Seriously, look at your closet and tell me you need another t-shirt, polo, shoes, bra, or whatever. If you have tags still on clothes, wear them.

For arguments sake, let's say you really "need" some new clothes. I would venture to say to skip the mall all together.

However, the big department stores can have some serious sales: up to 75% off plus an extra 20% off. Regardless of whether you shop at Dillard's® or JC Penny's® (notice I didn't say Nordstrom's® or the equivalent high-end department store), wait until they have these huge sales and then go look around. Be on guard though. These stores are here to make a sale and there is some serious science on how to manipulate us into buying things.

Stores know that if they mark down items at a high rate, put a time limit on it (this weekend only), and say all sales are final, you will experience pressure and regret if you pass up on item you were eyeballing. The major problem is that we will try on the pants and though they may be baggy or the shirt is slightly long in the arms, we justify buying it because the price is only $10 instead of $60. Don't do it. Once you get it home and your stress and excitement hormones have stabilized, you will try it on again and model for someone. Both of you will realize that it's not a perfect fit but will rationalize that it's ok and you still look "good enough." Try to avoid these situations.

Action tip: Stay calm at the store and don't buy just for the sake of buying. My rule of thumb is that if you don't feel more confident and attractive in it, don't buy it. Nothing is more of a waste of money than spending even a dime on a piece of clothing and then not actually wearing it. If you feel less than awesome and not spectacular when trying it on, skip the purchase.

Second idea for shopping for new clothes.

We have all seen the commercials to be a Maxxinista®, haven't we? Ross®, Marshal's®, Burlington®, and TJ Max® are all pretty much the same thing to me. They have either name brand clothes or boutique brands at discounted rates. Typically what they offer are last season's stuff that are leftover or sometimes a big brand will make an inferior quality product and sell directly to these stores. We can't really trust those marked down prices on the tags. Maybe some really were sold at $45 and now are $13, but that's a great big lie on many products. Regardless of the visual price manipulation, we can still shop here and get great deals. Lots of people enjoy the process of browsing. These stores, particularly for women, have ample supply of styles, variety, and even home décor for you to comb through. Guys have it much easier: you want polos, sweaters, t-shirts, or athletic gear? The same rules apply here as to the department stores. The difference is you need to set a price that you are willing to spend and stick to that. If you are unwilling to spend more than $16 for a new athletic polo then don't compromise for $20. If the perfect shirt is $19 and you can't find anything for $16, walk away and go to another store. Realistically, you probably don't really even need the item anyway. Sacrifice and delayed gratification are the mark of a sophisticated, intelligent adult and if you are in a financial crisis, it's time to step up your maturity.

Stores are experts at manipulation too. I'll use a grocery store as an example. Have you noticed the lingering smell of fresh bread when you walk into a big grocery store? It stimulates hunger and encourages you to buy more. Do you think all the dairy and meat are just randomly in the back of the store? Nope. You cross all the pretty fresh fruit and veggies first and then into all the aisles and aisles of processed, boxed, canned food. Profit margins are higher here because they last so long. A bag of chips and cereal is way more convenient than chopping up plums and peaches for a gourmet breakfast with eggs.

Cereals are laid out in a very specific manner that has real-world trial and error built in. The sugary name brand colorful boxes are exactly at the height of your little kid sitting in the cart and walking at your side. It's no wonder that lil' Adam was able to grab a leprechaun and then have an absolute meltdown because you told him to put it back. The healthier cereal is usually up high were adults can't even get to it and the off brand/ store brands are down below and sometimes next to the name brands. When shopping for cereal, especially if you have kids, buy the name brand once but don't throw away the box when done. Another option is to buy a rubber container that can fit 1.5 pounds of cereal and has a sealable flip top. Bring that home and have your kids pour the fancy brand into this container. Tell them you are making a change so that the cereal stays fresh and crispy longer. When that original is almost out, go back to the store and buy the own-brand cereal and refill the container. Figure something out to handle the kids questioning of the new shapes. From personal experience, I can say 7 out of 10 are really comparable in texture and flavor to the original. My disclaimer is that we should stop eating that sugary junk and don't feed it to our kids.

Between feeding our kids too much sugar, soda and, not exercising nearly enough, I'm quite frankly not shocked that parents think their kids are hyperactive. Do you remember how much time we played outside as kids during and after school? My parents would kick us outside in the hot Louisiana summer with a big jug of water and say, "Don't come back inside for a few hours."

Last bit of advice: De-Clutter

My clothes are old and have holes, you say. Really? Do they? Ok, I'll give you the benefit of the doubt. Throw them away, but that doesn't give you permission to get something new. People have written entire books on how to de-clutter your life. The closet purge will literally give you a sigh of relief and accomplishment when you are finished. While your first reaction will probably be reluctance and fear, it's a task worth doing.

I had a shopping spree and a dilemma a few years ago. I went to a big sale and bought $200 worth of dress clothes that averaged $11 per item. Those new items were on top of the stuff I already had. Did I need the new clothes? Yes and no, but it was a good choice for my professional image and I could afford it. One day I was reading one of those de-clutter books and went look at my wardrobe. I noticed I consistently only wore my favorite five or six shirts regularly and ignored the rest.

De-clutter books recommend a few things.

Step 1: Go through all your clothes and if there are stains, holes, broken zippers, or you haven't fit them in at least a year (I'm being generous on that time line) then it's time to throw them away. If the clothes that are too big or to thin are in good shape, donate them. Get a receipt for the donation and write that off your taxes.

Step 2: Ask yourself, your spouse, or a trusted friend to through your clothes with you go piece by piece and ask one question. Is this item fashionable? Some things might be old but are classic and others scream a decade ago. Get rid of the fashion faux pas. Hint: if you have ties or scarves that are older than three years old, they are probably out of style and they should be tossed. Do a quick search online for what's hot right now and pick up some new ones. Haven't we all made fun of the teacher with the gigantic 70s tie? Spend $10-20 and get a new tie or two.

Step 3: Now you should have cut down your closet. Say a prayer for peace, try transcendental meditation chants, or do whatever atheists do to calm down and re-center and move on. This step is all about figuring out what you actually wear.

Divide your closet with an obvious marker on a hanger. I used a suit because I rarely wear it and so it makes for a nice demarcation. After you wear an item and wash it, return it to the closet on the right side of the demarcation item (in my case, to the right of the suit). Do this for three to five months. Feel free to re-wear anything on the right as many times as you want. Just be honest and pick what you like and feel amazing in. After five months, you should see a clear distinction on what you do and you don't wear. Examine all the clothes on the left one more time and donate them because you are not wearing them. If you find yourself getting hung up on an item, hang on to it for another month and if you still haven't worn it, donate that too.

When I did this I realized I had a lot of sentimental t-shirts: favorite bands, Christian organization shirts, races, my alma mater gear, etc. I couldn't just throw away all those memories. The shirts were still in good shape. Some were worn and others were always a showcase novelty. I was stuck making a decision: keep my closet cluttered and unorganized or do something with them. After asking a few people their opinion, they afforded up an amazing and practical solution. Gather the shirts and have someone turn them into a quilt. Life Hack 101, boys and girls. I turned comfy, sentimental t-shirt graphics into a full-size quilt that I could display on a couch, guest bed, or snuggle with on a cold night. You are welcome!

I still use a demarcation item in my closet. These days, I wear everything on the left side of the item and once I run out of clean clothes on that side, I switch to the right. I like to cycle left and right because I can keep track of what I'm wearing and not wearing the same three shirts every week. Bonus, I am actually wearing all the clothes I own and therefore not wasting any of the money I spent on them. I suggest you cycle through all your clothes before re-wearing them.

Now you are done. How's it feel? Do you have a ton of closet space? Please do not run to the store to fill it back up. If you honestly need another dress shirt, or age appropriate blouse for work, maybe save for a month or two and get an updated one following the advice from earlier. Have fun shopping because you know you were smart and planned for the purchases. Be proud of yourself. You are growing.

Growth can hurt. When was the last time you grew as a person when everything was rainbows and ice cream on a hot day? Rarely, I know. The struggles in life are what stretch and challenge us to be better people. I hope you surround yourself with positive people and books and guard what you put into your mind. That way when challenges arise, you have the right mindset to overcome them.

New or Used Car

I've already touched on insurance so this section will focus on your actual car. Have you heard someone driving a luxury vehicle complain that the oil change and super premium gasoline is too much for them? Cry me a river, chump. If you can't afford the maintenance of your vehicle then get a normal car. I bought a sweet Mazda® Protégé 5® hatchback many years ago. That mere 120 hp engine was programmed to live up to the Zoom Zoom™ trademark. One thing I didn't realize about the car was the tire size. It was built to run on wide, low profile tires, which wear out faster and are more expensive to replace. Looking back, it wouldn't have changed my mind on the purchase but it sure did hit my wallet a few times.

When making a car purchase, you have to consider what the insurance will be on it. I'd rather not pay $300 a month for a turbo-charged car when the middle model is $150, but that's just me. I don't know where those extra 100 horses can roam in the urban jungle.

Something else to consider is the brand and model level. Just because you can afford a Lexus®, does it mean you should buy one? What about a high-level Toyota® with leather seats instead and save yourself $20,000? It's the nearly the same frame and engine. Again, this section is looking for ways to save you money. If you have a good salary and you are financially stable, then buy whatever your heart and wallet desires, especially if it falls into the proper percentage of your salary. If 10% of your salary only allows you to get a Honda® Civic® low end model, then you shouldn't buy the mid-level Acura®.

Another common concern is buying new or used. A used car that's just one year old costs about 20% less than new and a two-year old model is even cheaper. Let someone else take the drastic depreciation and you get a sweet deal. Of course, be wise about buying a used car. Don't get something that's quite old and in need of an engine belt replacement (100,000 miles) or worse, a transmission: if you can afford something better, that is.

The maintenance on a much older car cannot be ignored. Even if you saved a few thousand dollars on the front end, but every month you spend roughly $250 on repairs, then it won't take long to realize that you should have bought a newer model. Money exiting the bank account, time off work to fix the car, getting someone to pick you up, or spending your own time fixing it will all add up to more than you bargained for. Sometimes you have to consider what your time is worth as well as direct money spent.

These days, when you can get a brand new car at less than 3% interest but a bank loan for a used car at 5%, decisions start to get tougher. You can use an amortization calculator online to crunch the numbers to see which will save you money over a three-year payoff. I would still go out on a limb and say the two-year-old car with 30% depreciation will be more affordable. If a $15,000 car is 20% off then it costs $12,000, in case you aren't doing the math (30% is $10,500). Rates fluctuate all the time so if the rate is about the same, maybe go after a used model. Also, once the body shape changes (or generation) from one year to the next, the price really drops for that older body shape.

I'm not saying, "Save all your cash for 5 years then buy a used car and take on zero debt." If you are able to do that, you are awesome. Most of us don't have that willpower to save or the ability to do it. You still need to be saving =for a healthy size down payment. I'd recommend at least 10% saved plus tax, title and license, so let's say 15%. Since you will probably be financing a car, it's best to shop around banks and credit unions to get the best possible interest rate. Credit unions are an overlooked resource for banking and borrowing money.

What do you do if you have a car you can't afford and it's ruining you in every other area of life? Maybe it's time to cut your losses and sell it. You should contact an advisor on this issue to crunch the numbers. My thoughts are to find a car that fits with your approved income percentage for auto expenses.

How much do you owe on your car now? Can you sell it and pay the bank off or are you upside down on it? Can you afford the newly acquired used vehicle and the difference you owe to the bank from the first bad loan? Maybe you can talk to the bank and ask if they can spread that loss out over a year.

Here is my last word on how to make your car purchase even wiser and less expensive. Keep it as long as feasible. I haven't had very many cars in my life because I kept them 10-12 years. If my car has been paid off for five years and it's time to change the timing belt, I don't sweat that $1,000 because I'll be able to drive it for a few more years. Pay attention to the noises and how it drives over the years because you have to make a decision on fixing a transmission and driving it for many more years or selling it before it becomes a real issue.

That Mazda I bought was two years old and apparently that model year had a defect. At 80,000 miles, the transmissions on many of them broke. I purchased the extended warranty on it because it had more miles than normally driven in two years. You never know how the previous owner drove it. I won't advise you on whether you should get that warranty or not but use your gut. If I recall, that $3,000 repair didn't cost me a single penny more than the initial warranty. I guess I lucked out that it broke within the allotted time frame.

House

An often overlooked area of financial health is also the biggest asset: your home. This is arguably the most expensive purchase of your life and a decision that stays with you for 30 years. Well, that's how it used to be. Seems more and more people are moving around town, following jobs to new cities, and delaying that first purchase altogether. For some reason, our parents were capable of raising three kids in a 1,600 sq. ft. house or smaller, but my generation can't do without 2,200 sq. ft.+. I don't have an answer, unfortunately.

Personally I like the idea of the 900 sq. ft. or less tiny house, but it's impractical for a family. Companies have started to build these and I even saw a tiny home subdivision. It was so cute. Have you seen the variety of storage (shipping) container houses out there? Yes, the 20x10 metal structures that you can stack on a boat and ship across the ocean. They can be purchased at $2,000-5,000 apiece and you can have a crane put four of them in just the right spot for you. You can get super creative and have a sweet looking modern home with the crux of it being all storage containers. You have to wield, put sheet rock, plumbing, electricity, and all the normal stuff a house would need. After researching it, and having zero construction skills myself, I would be better off just buying some major developer's pre-fabricated. I've seen some 3,000 sq. ft. container homes that would at least make you appreciate it. Maybe that's the Colorado influence on me.

The housing market crash around 2007 was a rude awakening for just how overpriced a house can be. At the point of this book writing, most markets around the United States have balanced out and the housing prices are more accurate. Let's chat about a couple of the reasons why I think our homes have become a slight burden. In my opinion, we move around often because of new jobs in new cities and it can be difficult to stay in one house long enough to recoup all the real estate fees and closing costs. Also, many people have two kids and upgrade to a 2,200+sq. ft. house. I don't really care how big a house you think you need, my point is that every time you move, it's like restarting the clock on a 30-year mortgage. Hopefully you stayed at the first house long enough to pay some principle and are able to roll that into the next purchase. Sadly, I think that amount is quite small and the probability of paying a mortgage into retirement will be a strong possibility for most people. When you have to spend an extra $1,500 per month in retirement years for a house, it means you need to save even more when you are working. Another option is to downgrade to a condo or smaller home once you retire. Only buy what you need based on your lifestyle and family

I won't say what the right size home is for you because I obviously have no idea about your situation. If you are having some money issues and are looking for yet another way to lower your monthly expenses, then an evaluation of your living arrangement is necessary.

I grew up with a roommate, otherwise known as a younger brother. There is nothing wrong with sharing a room. When did it become so normal for each kid to have their own room? Sure, the kids need some privacy, but at what cost? Two beds or bunk beds and two desks so they can do homework are functionally all they need. They can watch TV and play on the internet in the living room or have another area so you can monitor what they watch and still enjoy your programs too.

Is it time to downgrade from what you live in now? I know we can get sentimental over the house mom and dad lived before the divorce. Maybe it's sentimental because you both raised your kids in this house and it would be too painful to leave. I get it and you have the right to not want to change those memories. Really, you aren't abandoning those memories because you can look at pictures and replay those memories in your mind.

On the other hand, if you have a 2,500 sq. ft. house and your kids are gone, maybe the maintenance of the house is becoming too much to handle and you are nearing retirement. What's the problem with a downgrade? A smaller house could be a golden nugget to get you out of debt at any age. Imagine dropping your mortgage by 34%. What could you do with that extra income?

Condos can be a great idea. Some experts will say they aren't a good investment for resale, but that is dependent on your area of the country. I bought a condo in Colorado for a steal because it wasn't in the best division, even though it was nestled next to some average ones. Five years later, I nearly doubled my original investment and rolled it into a new home. Talk to a realtor and they can help you plan which neighborhoods are available, school districts, condos vs. smaller homes and will give you sound advice to consider before ever going out and look at homes.

When you hear that a house is 1,500 sq. ft., what comes to mind? Small, cramped, just right, endless possibilities, or is it hard to imagine at all? Since I have leased space for a business and have seen many of my colleagues' offices, I can confidently say the perceived space of 1,500 sq. ft. is based solely on how it is built out. We've all been to a house that looks huge on the inside and one that seems very boxy and square. That is because of interior design. Maybe the space would feel larger if the ceiling was a foot higher or the kitchen and living room were only separated by an open sitting bar counter / island instead of a wall.

My parents had three kids in a 1300 sq. ft. home so they decided to close in the garage and gain 500 sq. ft. Living in the heat of South Louisiana allowed us kids to have a huge air conditioned play room. Twenty years later and after three other people owned that home, it went up for sale. One previous owner decided to convert the playroom into a master bedroom and linen area. That house now has four bedrooms and two baths and if it wasn't for the poor craftsmanship and unfinished work on the upgrade, it probably would have sold for a lot more money.

Have you ever had the idea of adding an enclosed outdoor

patio off the house? What about enclosing the garage or if you live in the right part of the world, finishing the basement? Those two options are cheaper to build than an official house extension and will add more room and depth of space for your enjoyment. The benefits don't end at aesthetics either. A finished basement compared to a dusty boring one, although not valued the same as the main house, will increase the overall house price. A friend of mine (who did the work himself) added a trendy master bath, closet, bedroom, entertainment room complete with an elliptical machine, and walled off the utility area all in the basement. He literally doubled the living area of his house. A side bonus is he can pretty much just live downstairs, and when guests are over, the main house looks clean and tidy.

Renting an apartment or a house might be a good option for you too. Maybe you despise outdoor maintenance or only plan to live in an area for less than five years. One good reason to rent is when you are new to an area and want to get to know it before picking a neighborhood. I've known more than a few people who live in an area because of a "school district" but then realize that almost everything they do is across town, near schools with a near identical school report card. That's a lot of wasted time in traffic. This could have been avoided if they rented for 6-12 months first. More often than not, however, renting ends up costing more than mortgage repayment which makes it hard for me to recommend renting.

There are times in life, whether from bad credit or not having enough savings for the down payment or the credit score available to purchase a house, when you just have to rent. Just make a wise choice when signing a lease. Do you get a pool or a gym with your apartment building? If you do, that means you can save money on memberships. Just food for thought.

Charity Donations

We see tragedies on our Facebook feeds every day: from terrorist attacks to insane natural disasters like out of control fires and hurricanes that wreak havoc on multiple states. We have kids who want to go to college but need financial assistance. Schools that can't afford books and basic supplies for ten year olds. Police and firefighters who cook barbeques and raise money to supplement what taxes can't cover. Church attendees who spread their faith by helping the local community via tithes. Organizations that need your help to stop deadly diseases from spreading in foreign countries. Organizations fighting to stop sex slavery and child trafficking. Groups who build water wells, buy a dairy cow, chickens, or even a sewing machine for a village so they can make money. You can even support political groups of your choosing with the hope that your viewpoints will be better represented. With so many options to donate and be charitable, I'm sure you could find something to get behind and support with your hard-earned money. In the following paragraphs, let's discuss some of the other reasons why you might consider spending your money on others.

Unless you think giving taxes to the government is your version of donations, most of us understand that giving money to official charities allows us to reduce our yearly taxes. There is an upper limit of how much you can reduce your taxes by charitable donations each year so Google® it or ask an accountant. Some of you may want to give up to that amount to maximize the savings.

I've focused so far on money donations, but don't forget that your time is the most valuable asset you actually have. With all the callings of life, you probably don't have a lot of time to spend doing the things you really want to do much less help out strangers. This is why volunteering is such a blessing to organizations. They know you could be playing with your kids, or creating a side hustle business project, but instead you choose to clean the poop out of the dog shelter or canvas the neighborhood, pick up trash, or lick stamps for your political cause. Why do you think volunteers get t-shirts? It's not just for easy recognition of who is in charge but it's also a "reward" for spending your time with them. I can speak for my own organization efforts; a volunteer is the lifeblood of the organization and we thank them all for their time from the bottom of our hearts.

Studies have found that retirees who volunteer actually live longer. Not only does it give them something to do after retiring from 20-30 years at a 9-5 job, it gives them a sense of purpose, drive, and a renewed reason to live. For us working age folks, volunteering time or money makes you feel good about yourself. You know you just helped a family of four pay the bills that month. You just helped a 30-year-old widow in a poor foreign country get a sewing machine that she can now use to feed her two kids and fix the leak in her roof. That $10 a month paid for a kid to finish high school and land a job that can support his entire extended family. You and your family mowed the lawn of five families' gardens who, for whatever reason, are unable to physically do that anymore.

We know all the people we helped are grateful, but really, it turns out that the person we may have helped the most mentally is ourselves. A sense of good accomplishment and less selfishness is a nice break from the negative cycle that so many find themselves in. You might just find giving of your time and money is a nice stress relief too.

Another great benefit of giving time is that it can build friendships with a wide array of people and it prevents feelings of loneliness developing. It makes you more gracious for what you have. A common statement from people who go on a mission trip to a poor country is that they have a greater appreciation for the things they have, the country they live in, and what their parents have given them. Is it any wonder that when business tycoons like Bill Gates and Warren Buffett have gotten older and established, they switched their focus to a more lasting legacy, i.e. setting up charitable foundations?

For those who don't trust churches but also realize that many organizations spend money poorly, you can search online for sites that rank major charitable organizations. These sites can break down how much of your dollar is spent on administration, advertising, and how much is spent on the purpose and mission of the organization. I won't bad mouth any by name here, but I can think of two major ones that have notoriously low rates of money going to the cause versus the higher-ups' mega paychecks. I'm not saying they shouldn't be paid nicely to manage millions of donations, just that it seems counterintuitive to be compensated like big-wig bankers and investment hedge managers.

Sorry, bank employees. We can't afford to give you adequate health insurance because of our shareholder responsibilities. Wait, didn't your top executives make multi-million dollar bonuses. Couldn't the company have said, let's just spend $100 million of our $1.5 billion profit to take care of our employees? In a couple years, the stock will balance out and the reputation we garnered will outshine the initial cost layout. Wishful thinking, right? I don't think the government has the right to dictate how much profit a company can make, but at what point does a company have an obligation, if ever, to take better care of their employees? Could it be a percentage of profit over $500 million or a sliding scale based on factors that are above their own pay grade to understand? Some manufacturing company owners would still dump all their toxic waste byproducts into the nearest river if it wasn't for government oversight. I read an article about a company doing just that despite that country's laws forbidding it. Rant over.

Like it or not, donating money is also a biblical topic with a fancy word called tithing. I'm not going to quote scripture to you, but the topic (money) is covered many times in the bible. There's a saying, "I don't have to follow you around to know what you care about most, just show me your bank statements." Some of us have been burned in the past by cheating pastors and have sworn to never trust one again. That is an interesting way to live life, in my opinion. I have had bad experiences at certain chain restaurants but have still gone back to a different location. I've even had a bad dental experience and just found a new one next time for a cleaning. Regardless, tithing is a principle held not just in Christian circles but in all religions I'm aware of. While living in China and visiting lots of ancient Buddhist temples, I saw people giving fruit, cakes, fake money, and purchasing blessed/prayed over jade pendants and bracelets. Since they are recommended by the monk in the temple, the price is nearly triple what you would purchase it for at the local jewelry shop.

A tithe is technically 10% of your net income (after taxes), but the bible also says to give with a cheerful heart. I'm no expert but if we are guilt tripped into it or feel resentful for giving 10% then it's best to give what you are willing to give with happy feelings. Feeling manipulated and resentful is not the type of heartfelt giving God is talking about. Be a cheerful giver, whether that's 3% or even $50. For argument sake, let's say you subscribe to the 10% rule, but you just really have strange feelings about giving that kind of money to one church. Maybe they spent it poorly in the past or you make so much money that you can't trust one church with $100,000 or you've been taken advantage of and you just aren't comfortable donating more than 3%. One way to look at it: you attend service, benefit from a pastor, air conditioning, paved parking lot, and they do help the community so some percentage is reasonable to give back. What do you do with the other 7%? Go back to the first paragraph of this topic and look at all the organizations just hoping to get a piece of your income pie.

Many charities have zero religious affiliations and many do have a core belief in serving the faith you subscribe to. You could probably contact your own church, synagogue, or whatever and ask for a faith-based group that does whatever activity you find most deserving and feel passionate about. I could support a foundation looking to dig water wells in Africa that has a Christian mission or one that does it purely for the humanitarian efforts—the choice is ours. Personally, I believe in giving to Christian organizations of varying styles and some going to my local place of worship. My contribution helps out my own community and has a global reach.

Basics on Retirement

Let me be honest from the start about retirement. I'm not an expert in any form, but I do enjoy reading and listening to podcasts about investing though I'm not really offering any strong opinions. One strong opinion, however, is that you need to seek expert advice and you need to save for retirement.

Talk to someone and they will gladly have you take a quick assessment of your risk tolerance and tailor make recommendations for your unique situation. They will also be able to give you a realistic amount of savings you would need to maintain the quality of life that you live now and not out live your savings. You can look at your local bookstore or on Amazon® and you will see thousands of books on the subject. One theme that comes up all the time is to not try and time the stock market. Sure, you hear about a few people who have made money timing the market but you know what they don't mention? Like a gambler at a casino, the stock market timer is seldom going to tell you that they lost 80% of their money last week. They just tell about when they made 125% profit in one day. Do yourself a favor and go in for the long haul. Buying a mutual fund and holding it for 20 years is typically what people recommend. The experts will typically choose where to invest for you so don't stress about the thousands of options.

Personally, I'm a big fan of low cost, low fee index funds. Over 25 years, they tend to outperform actively managed funds. Actively managed funds buy and sell way more often and incur more fees. Even if both styles of funds, index vs. actively managed, were to make the exact same return on investment (profit as a percentage), the index would still win because of lower fees. From what I've gathered over the years, actively managed funds might outperform for a few years but they inevitably slow down. In fact, they might have a good few years and then horrible years to come. Many don't even exist after 10 years.

I know you have heard of the phrase diversify. Diversify, or diversification, means you spread your money out by buying different types of companies and funds. You don't want to have your entire retirement tied up in one company and then that company goes bankrupt. Now you are left with no profit and you lost the initial investment. That's what a mutual fund combats so well. They will have shares of say 300 different companies so that if one is not doing well, they can sell it and buy some other company that is succeeding. It balances the losers with the winners and the status quo companies. You can buy funds of USA companies, Asia companies, European companies, companies expected to grow fast or slow, funds that only buy stock in companies for energy, oil, food, and the list goes on and on. If you have a preference for what to invest in, just tell your advisor and they can give you their opinion.

Pick a good advisor. Find out how long they have worked in the industry and with one company. I've seen so many bounce from one company to the next and others that don't last three years in the business. One thing is for certain, they make money based on what you invest. Regardless of whether you make 30% one year and -20% the next, if you put $10,000 in their hands, they get a percentage of that. Maybe if their pay was tied more to results, we wouldn't have so many greedy advisors selling us products that benefit them more than you. Some companies have their own funds and unsurprisingly, the sales force recommends them more than any other. Because investing is a profitable business, the higher ups can run promotions to their employees to sell a certain amount of XYZ fund and the salesman gets a bonus based on how much money they can bring into that exact fund. Would you be surprised if suddenly XYZ fund became the top five seller this month during such a promotional period when it is normally ranked at 30?

There are plenty of honest, hard-working advisors that want nothing more than to see you succeed for retirement. They only work for respectable companies that have their customers' best interest at heart. Companies like Wealthfront®, Vanguard®, and even Edward Jones® are good places to start. I know plenty of independent companies that have amazing advisors too. They have access to almost all the same funds as these big name places like Prudential®, Principle®, TD Ameritrade®, and Fidelity®. Don't be afraid to use a smaller company just because they don't spend millions a year advertising on TV and sponsoring football games. Again though, do your homework so you don't pick an unethical, Ponzi scheme, embezzling joker of an advisor. Call around and ask for a referral of current clients to see if they are satisfied. Especially consider asking for someone who has been with them for a long time and are actually in retirement.

What's the golden rule of investing?

- If it sounds too good to be true, it probably is
- Don't be greedy
- Buy when the price is low and sell when the price is high.
- Try not to watch too much cable TV about stock market topics. They need to find and perhaps embellish stories because they have air time to fill every night. Sensational topics make good news, crazy, right?

Roth IRA

A Roth IRA is money you can invest after taxes. The biggest perk is that the money grows over your lifetime and there is no extra tax when you finally pull it out in retirement. Every year, the rules change but as of 2016, here are the basics. If you are single and make less than $132,000, you can invest up to $5,500. If you are married and file jointly, you can make up to $194,000 and invest $5,500 each. There is a lot more to them than this, like rules on how to withdraw money early and the penalties incurred, but you can buy a book on that.

Traditional IRA

The Traditional IRA has a $5,500 contribution limit per person per year. The perk of this investment style is that the money invested lowers your taxable income for that year. The drawback is that when you take money out during retirement, that money is taxed at the current year's tax rate. There is a lot more to them than this, like rules on how to withdraw money early and the penalties incurred, but you can also buy a book on that.

401K/ Simple IRA

These types of retirement accounts can be set up as a Roth or Traditional. The major difference is that these are employee-based plans. You can contribute up to $18,000 a year and your employer will match anywhere from 1-3%. That employer is literally just giving you money so why not at least invest the same percentage that they match.

Trust Fund

Maybe you heard of a trust fund baby. That usually has a negative connotation of a college kid who campaigns against corporate greed and the wrongs of the world and backpacks around Europe but is secretly wealthy and doesn't have to worry about money because of their parents set up a trust fund for them. So what is a trust fund? Well, it's a legal document that can protect money you earned for future generations. A lawyer can set up a trust fund document in many different ways. The easiest way for me to write about this is to provide examples.

A basic family without a lot of wealth could set one up in case the parents died and the life insurance policy payout would go to a young kid. Obviously, a 10-year-old child isn't able to handle $1,200,000. Plus, who ever raises them will need some help too. A trust document can outline where the money goes: a bank, a non-retirement IRA so it can grow with the stock market, etc. Then they plan the detail, such as when the kid turns 18, some of the money can be used for high education or trade school. At 25, a sum of money is released and they can use it for a house down payment or whatever they want at this point. Some might even not give the child full control until the age of 30, when they can have a job, a family, an education, and are more mature and able to handle finances. Last thing you want is your kid to "win the life insurance lottery" and dive deep into drugs and alcohol like lottery winners and childhood actors have been shown to do.

Maybe you have a disabled child, so you set up a trust fund so all their needs are met when you do finally die. That might mean a facility, high costs drugs, and many other options.

If a family is really rich, and they want a company or their wealth to benefit generations to come, they can set it up so that the inheritance is paid out by only a certain amount per year, or just the interest earned on the money. Now that original nest egg can be guaranteed to last forever.

Buying Houses

I won't go into too many details about this style of retirement because there are tons of seminars and books you can study on it. With that caveat, real estate can be a great retirement vehicle, or at least a piece of your retirement package. The idea is to buy houses below market value, fix them up enough so they can be rented, and then have a renter pay the mortgage. The house, condo etc. might make you $100-300 profit each month. After 10-20 years, the house is paid off and now you have an extra $800 each month. Well, if you started buying one house every few years since you were 30, you potentially could have 11 houses. If each generates even $600 a month, that's $6,600 a month just from real estate. There are lots of pitfalls to be weary of but it can be worth it. Obviously, if a tenant destroys your house, you have to repair it and if you can't rent it then you still have to cover the payments. If you suddenly have four houses with a mortgage and no one renting them, you could be in dire financial strain in a hurry. Study hard, get some mentors and this could be a viable option for some people.

Rapid Compounding Debt Payoff

For some people, this next section will be new and mind blowing. Different 'talking heads' have trademarked a term for it, but really its rapid compounding debt payoff. There are generally two ways of performing this rapid payoff: paying off the highest interest rate first or smallest balance first. It's my opinion that the latter is best. By paying off the smallest balance first, you quickly get a sense of accomplishment that will motivate you to continue to sacrifice and be smart with your payoff and not accumulate more debt.

Steps for Rapid Compounding Debt Payoff

1. Gather all your credit cards, car loans, boat loans, loans from your momma, etc.
2. Write down the name of the cards, the dollar amount balance and the interest rate. The order is not important at this point; just jot them all down for easy comparison.
3. Now arrange them on the paper again with the lowest

amount listed first.
4. Make sure you are currently paying the minimum balance on all your debt. The last thing you want is to get non-payment and late fees.
5. Next up is hitting the lowest balance (not the lowest interest rate) with as much money as you can. That means if you were normally paying the minimum on all your cards but paying an extra $50 on one, then that $50 will now be put to the lowest balance and only pay the minimum on the other ones for now.
6. You can use some of the tactics I've written about to free up some money (remember an example is cutting cable and buying Hulu so you free up $75) and put that toward your lowest balance. Sometimes your lowest balance is still quite high, so hang in there. Put extra money toward it each month and don't stop until it hits zero.
7. Time goes by and suddenly it is paid off. CELEBRATE! You did an amazing thing, take a moment to really enjoy and relish your accomplishment.
8. Here's where even more self-discipline comes into play. Now, every single penny you were paying on that debt goes to the next lowest debt. Don't be tempted to give up or, worse, keep only paying the minimum balance on the rest of your debt or, even worse, start spending that money on frivolous stuff.
9. Example: first debt you managed to pay $175 per month and the next lowest was a minimum of $30. Since you finished Debt One, now you put that $175 on top of the $30 minimum payment of Debt Two. Now you are putting $205 a month on the balance.
10. Once that one is done, repeat the process.
11. Following the example: take the $205 per month on Debt

Two and add it to the next minimum payment for Debt Three. If Debt Three was $70 per month minimum, now you are paying $275 a month. Eventually, you get through all the debt.
12. Congrats on getting debt free.
13. Don't be fooled: if you are neck deep in debt, this process could literally take years.

CONCLUSION

Throughout this book, I have introduced new ideas and blueprints to get stronger, extend your cardiovascular exercise, make better food choices and even how to strengthen the nervous system. Be gentle with yourself. We all fall off the wagon, straight up cheat, or quit for a while. My big suggestion and encouragement is to be patient with yourself. If you do cheat, accept it and move on. The next meal and the next day are always a reset. You ate two pieces of cheesecake, you quit the treadmill in 5 minutes instead of going your goal of 12... alright. That was today, but just push reset and stick to your goals tomorrow. I really hope that my explanations made it simple for you to visualize yourself implementing everything. A small step today builds each day until one day, maybe 4 -6 months from now, you step on the scale and have lost 20 pounds, are doing 30 minutes of continuous cardio and no longer crave carb-tastic buffet lines. My hope for you is to achieve your health goals and if my advice has helped you, then this book was worth writing. Please search for me on all social media and let me know how things are going.

I gave you a lot of information to process. Go back and reread it a few times. Explore what others have written on some of these topics to get a full picture of what is in store for you. I just ask that you do something. Reading and doing math are a fun use of time but reading and implementing are two different things. If you expect to see changes in your blood work, thighs and waist line, you have to take action.

One of my goals is to appeal to those who ask, "What do I need to do. I will do it immediately" and to others who ask, "I can't just jump in fully committed. Is there a way to tip toe into this and finally be fully engaged?" I hope giving you options, allowing for mistakes, and starting slow gives you the encouragement to get started. I know you can do it because I was once where you are. It takes small steps to see improvements in health, food choices, and exercise, but today's choices turn into tomorrow's health.